Exploring the Interconnected Complexities of COVID-19

Exploring the Interconnected Complexities of COVID-19

By

Keekok Lee

Cambridge
Scholars
Publishing

Exploring the Interconnected Complexities of COVID-19

By Keekok Lee

This book first published 2023

Cambridge Scholars Publishing

Lady Stephenson Library, Newcastle upon Tyne, NE6 2PA, UK

British Library Cataloguing in Publication Data
A catalogue record for this book is available from the British Library

ISBN (10): 1-5275-2532-5
ISBN (13): 978-1-5275-2532-0

CONTENTS

ACKNOWLEDGEMENTS

I would like to thank Anthony Leggett for his insightful comments and suggestions for improvement. Flaws still remain, and I am sure that many do; however, they are entirely my own responsibility.

Professor Leggett has also kindly agreed to write a Forward for the book, for which many thanks yet again.

FOREWORD

ANTHONY J. LEGGETT

In this slim and unpretentious volume, the author deploys her encyclopaedic knowledge of Chinese and Western traditions in both philosophy and medicine to place the history of the COVID-19 pandemic and efforts to combat it in a wider philosophical and sociological context. In particular she emphasizes the contrast between the more "clinical" and individualistic approach of most Western nations with the more "epidemiological" and communitarian attitudes adopted in most of the East Asian cultural sphere.

Whether or not they agree with her conclusions, readers will acquire a refreshingly different perspective on the pandemic from that which they are liable to pick up from much of the Anglo-Saxon media.

CHAPTER 1

LAYING OUT THE INTERCONNECTED THEMES FOR EXPLORATION

This book necessarily crosses disciplines as it is primarily an exploration of COVID-19 as epidemic and pandemic from the vantage point of the philosophy of disease/illness. Philosophy of medicine, thus conceived, necessarily covers the Humanities, the Social Sciences, the Life Sciences and the Health Sciences.

A lot is now known of the science of the disease, known as COVID-19, since its first appearance just over three years ago. The World Health Organisation/WHO as well as the *Lancet* have published their reports on it. What has not been done is a systematic attempt to analyse the phenomenon from the standpoint of the philosophy of disease/illness as it affects individuals and society. To do justice to the scope of the information and data, this philosophy of disease/illness must address itself not only to the issues arising from the natural sciences, such as biology, genetics, bacteriology, clinical medicine, epidemiology but must also concern itself with those arising from the social sciences, such as economics, sociology, politics, geopolitics. This means that the different strategies of coping with the epidemic/pandemic must also be contextualised in terms of the "ideological" differences between cultures and societies. In other words, the nature of a disease/illness such as COVID-19 must be understood not only in terms of objective/scientific facts but also in the inescapably value-ladenness of medicine itself, especially in a pandemic. One needs also to explore a core issue, the competing causal models. Two are identified – one which is monofactorial and where the causal arrow is unidirectional, while the other is multifactorial and where the causal arrow is bidirectional. These two models underpin respectively, by and large, the two main domains of modern medicine, Clinical Medicine and Epidemiology. Exploring them would enable one to unravel some of the complexities behind COVID-19.

This book, in the first instance, attempts to explore the nature of COVID-19 through posing the following questions:

1. What could be said to be the cause of the illness?

2. Who is likely to be infected?
3. Where is infection likely to take place?
4. When is infection likely to occur?

It will demonstrate that the four Ws listed above are interconnected (IC); that interconnectedness may be summed up as the 4**W**s+IC formula. In turn, it will show that these themes are the very ones which preoccupy biomedicine today under its two main domains of investigation, namely, Clinical Medicine and Epidemiology. However, Epidemiology is standardly portrayed as "substandard" while Clinical Medicine is put on a pedestal marked "superior" and "methodologically impeccable/privileged". [1] The book aims to challenge this standard assessment of the two domains. Indeed, it argues that the causal model underlying Clinical Medicine (standardly theorised) is too simplistic and that which underpins Epidemiology is more adequate to account for medical data and evidence, across the board. In other words, Epidemiology, far from being the "pariah" should, instead, be the standard-bearer of "scientificity" in all domains of Medical Thinking. The notion of vaccines will be explored to further bring out the interconnectivity between the two domains of Clinical Medicine on the one hand and Epidemiology on the other. It will argue that Epidemiological Thinking is Ecosystem Thinking and that Ecosystem-nesting is an appropriate analytical tool to shed light on all domains of medicine. This way of looking puts paid to the Monogenic Conception of Disease which has, since its inception in the 1890s, over roughly seven decades, powerfully impacted Clinical Medicine. (See Chapter 2.)

Furthermore, the book will excavate and bring to light the values underpinning all the themes to be examined, especially with regard to how different countries/cultures respond to COVID-19. It will use mask-wearing as a case study to explore some of these differences in the core values embedded in two prominent yet different cultural/philosophical traditions in the world, namely, the modern Western (since the seventeenth century)

---

[1] This disparity has remarkably been commented upon by Mahbubani 2022. Mahbubani is a retired Singapore diplomat and now a renowned scholar of geopolitics. However, he has put his finger on the right spot in his comments on the COVID-19 pandemic, one of which reads: "The second way was to focus on biomedicine, with its focus on individual behavior, instead of social medicine. But understanding individual behavior is not enough to counter epidemics like COVID -19 that spread faster if we don't take care of social conditions." (Mahbubani, 2022, 248)

on the one hand and the Chinese on the other (often said to be at least three thousand years old). [2]

Chapter 2 (**The Cause of COVID-19 is SARS-CoV-2, or Is It?**) examines the following issues:

(a) Why it appears so "natural" to pick on the virus, SARS-CoV-2 as the cause of COVID-19. Can this ease be explained simply in terms of the historical contributions of medical giants such as Pasteur and Koch, under whose impetus the Monogenic Conception of Disease was formulated?
(b) It looks at the phenomenon of infected people who are asymptomatic to see if the Monogenic Conception of Disease could do justice to it. This phenomenon occurs in other cases of infectious diseases such as peptic ulcer disease, even though the infectious agent in this case is not a virus, but a bacterium, *H. pylori*.
(c) In other words, to pose the question: What could be said to be the relevant set of causal factors of COVID-19 or of peptic ulcer disease? [3] is more appropriate than posing the more simplistic question: What is the cause of COVID-19 or of peptic ulcer disease?

Chapter 3 (**Who Manifests a Disease? A Cut-and-Dry Matter?**) continues to test the validity of the Monogenic Conception of Disease by investigating how well it might fare in another context of disease-generation, when the relevant item is said to be a gene. It is tested against the disease called Phenylketonuria, said to be caused by a single defective gene. The conclusion of this exploration confirms the design flaw of the Monogenic Conception of Disease. Phenylketonuria is adequately diagnosed and treated by acknowledging the relevance both of the defective gene and a set of adverse environmental factors, that the one without the other would fail to bring on the disease. In other words, the **W**ho question, like the **W**hat question is adequately answered only in terms of the complex relationships between a factor studied in labs under Clinical Medicine as well as certain relevant factors in the environment studied by Epidemiology.

Chapter 4 (**Spatial-temporal Aspects of Disease-generation: The Where and When Questions**) tests the Monogenic Conception of Disease yet again, this time in the context of the **W**here question, to show that the flaw of the conception lies in ignoring the kind of issues raised by it. The **W**here question brings to the fore the relevance of Epidemiology to the

---

[2] While the Western tradition is traced back to ancient Greece, the Chinese is usually taken to be represented by the ethical thinking of Confucius (c 551 – c 479 BCE).

[3] See Mackie, 1965, 245-65; also, Chapter 5 of this book.

understanding of disease-generation and disease-transmission of a pathogenic virus, like SARS-CoV-2. At the same time, it also acknowledges the contribution of Clinical Medicine in understanding the transmission of a disease like COVID-19. In other words, it is through the joint effort of Clinical Medicine and Epidemiology that we can hope to understand and control the disease. This chapter, therefore, may also be understood as an attempt to answer the **W**hen question – a disease will become an epidemic and/or a pandemic when the relevant causal conditions happen to obtain within a certain segment(s) of the population, such as the elderly especially those with co-morbidities who are also vaccine-hesitant.

Chapters 2, 3 and 4 can be said to be dedicated to exploring the Monogenic Conception of Disease for two reasons: (a) from the standpoint of the history of medicine, given its powerful impact on Clinical Medicine for several decades (1876-1968), to show where its limitations lie in the context of the SARS-CoV-2/COVID-19 epidemic/pandemic and (b) also thereby, to challenge the orthodox understanding between Clinical Medicine (deemed superior) on the one hand and Epidemiology (deemed inferior) on the other. Furthermore, the book makes a distinction (in these chapters and throughout the book) between two versions of the Monogenic Conception of Disease: it calls one the Classical Version (or the non-dogmatic version) and the other, the dogmatic version.[4] It argues that Robert Koch, an acknowledged pioneer of the Age of Bacteriology failed to make such a distinction unambiguously, thereby muddying the waters.

The clarification of these matters then permits the book to move on to the next chapter. Chapter 5 (**"The Cause" in Terms of Controllability and Preventability**) examines Collingwood's Sense II of Cause, which singles out as "the cause" a factor in Mackie's account (as explored in Chapter 2) in terms of what he calls the "inus conditions". While Mackie's account is relevant to an explanatory context of disease/illness, Collingwood's is pertinent to the practical context of controlling a disease in the population. As such it cuts across the Clinical Medicine-Epidemiology divide, as an effective measure could either be a pharmaceutical (Clinical Medicine) or a non-pharmaceutical (Epidemiological) intervention.

Chapter 6 (**COVID-19, Vaccines and Vaccination: What they teach us about the nature of Medicine, Illness and Society**) in elaboration with

---

[4] The dates mentioned – 1876 to 1968 – are chosen for the following reasons: Koch's first pronouncement on the germ theory occurred in a paper he delivered in 1876. As we shall see, Stewart 1968 published in *The Lancet* his view that the germ theory had by 1968 (90 years after its first pronouncement) become a dogma. The critique of the Monogenic Conception of Disease undertaken in this book is, indeed, from the vantage point that it might have assumed the status of a dogma.

Chapter 5 focusses on the concept of vaccines and vaccination in order to further demonstrate that the Clinical Medicine-Epidemiology divide is unsustainable and flawed, as it is unintelligible when contextualised in either domain alone. The nature of medicine/disease/illness must be understood as being situated within society in general, and more, specifically within the different strata or classes into which society is divided. By so doing, it also challenges the highest level of probity bestowed on Clinical Medicine at the expense of Epidemiology which is considered to play the role of "Cinderella" to it as Epidemiology, given its nature, is incapable of satisfying the methodological requirements of the Randomised Controlled Trial.

Chapter 7 (**Ecosystem Thinking is Epidemiological Thinking Which is Medical Thinking**) explores in some detail the concept of Ecosystem Thinking, advanced by the author, in terms of Ecosystem-nesting in order to bring out clearly the Wholist [5] orientation of Medical Thinking in all domains. The concept of Ecosystem Thinking is advocated as an appropriate analytical research tool which can also be used outside the sphere of medicine, as it is primarily a version of Systems Thinking.

Chapter 8 (**COVID-19 and Mask-wearing: In the Context of Geopolitical and Other Values**) focusses, in the main, on mask-wearing in order to explore COVID-19 in the context of geopolitics. It explores the values embedded in the ideology of the West, as instantiated by the USA on the one hand and on the other, that of China. It proposes a spectrum with High Individualism/HI (the US) at one end and Low Individualism/LI (China) at the other. This in turn raises the issue of the relationship between Classical Liberalism with High Individualism on the one hand and Low Individualism, on the other, with some surprising conclusions. It also leaves space to discuss the relationship between self and other(s) respectively under the two versions of Individualism.

The chapter also looks briefly at another epidemiological measure which has been highly criticised by High Individualism – it is the lockdown. It shows yet again that in contrast to the high individualist vantage point, the non-pharmaceutical strategy of controlling COVID-19 via the lockdown is perfectly compatible with Low Individualism or even more strongly could be shown to be derived from its metaphysics of Wholism within which philosophical framework Epidemiological Thinking is embedded.

Chapter 9 (**Conclusion: Interconnectedness and Wholism**) maintains that the book has established, in the main, the following theses:

---

[5] This author prefers to use "Wholist" and "Wholism" instead of the more usual "Holism" for the obvious reason that the former terms make it clear that they are semantically linked with the term "whole". They also capture the ontological status of the concept behind the words better than "Holism".

(a) The Monogenic Conception of Disease (held as dogma) is tested in the context of the SARS-CoV-2/COVID-19 epidemic and pandemic of the last three or so years and found to be untenable yet again. This conclusion shows the need to distinguish the Classical Version of the Monogenic Conception of Disease from the version which holds it as dogma.
(b) The causal model in Medical Thinking is not monofactorial and unidirectional but multifactorial and reciprocal/bidirectional (with feedback mechanisms.
(c) It looks at Mackie's analysis of cause in terms of "inus conditions" as well as Collingwood's in terms of controllability or preventability in order to show where their respective insights lie.
(d) The above if correct would undermine the usual division in biomedicine into two domains, Clinical Medicine and Epidemiology, with the latter perceived as "inferior" to the former, as Epidemiology cannot satisfy certain evidential and methodological requirements that the former is capable of doing.
(e) The concept of vaccines and vaccination is explored to show that it cannot be properly grasped unless understood as having a foot in either of these two domains.
(f) The concept of Ecosystem Thinking in terms of Ecosystem-nesting is a more comprehensive research analytical tool to grasp both Clinical Medicine and Epidemiology within a single philosophical-causal framework. Such a framework can do better justice to the complex interconnectedness of the four leading questions which this book has called the 4**W**s+IC formula, that is to say, in the generation of disease/illness in society, there are four interrelated aspects to be explored, namely, the **W**hat, **W**ho, **W**hen and **W**here dimensions.
(g) Ecosystem Thinking/Ecosystem-nesting also brings out clearly the value-ladenness of all forms of Medical Thinking including geopolitical values in a pandemic such as COVID-19.
(h) In addition, it briefly explores the concept of Wholism, its emphasis on the interconnectedness of its constituent parts thereby giving rise to properties which are more than the sum of the properties of its parts, as well as its underlying values which underpin Epidemiological Thinking as Medical Thinking.

CHAPTER 2

THE CAUSE OF COVID-19 IS SARS-COV-2, OR IS IT?

This chapter examines the following issues:

1. Why does it appear so "natural" to pick on the virus, SARS-CoV-2 as the cause of COVID-19?
2. Can this ease be explained simply in terms of the historical contributions of medical giants such as Pasteur and Koch, under whose impetus the Monogenic Conception of Disease was formulated?
3. Is there an alternative viable criterion of selecting a set of several relevant variables as "the cause" of a disease/an illness?
4. In other words, this chapter is an attempt to answer the **W**hat question by arguing that to pose the question: What could be said to be the relevant set of causal factors of COVID-19? is more appropriate than posing the simplistic question: What is the cause of COVID 19? and to answer it in terms of SARS-CoV-2.

The Monogenic Conception of Disease

The Monogenic Conception of Disease is based on the pioneering work of two giants, Louis Pasteur (1822-1895) and Robert Koch (1843-1910) which ushered in modern Western medicine, today called biomedicine, or more specifically the prestigious branch of it called Clinical Medicine. The conception of disease replaced the ancient paradigm of the Four Humours handed down by Ancient Greek culture.[1] Pasteur's work on microbiology

---

[1] Humours in this context refer to bodily fluids (blood, yellow bile, black bile and phlegm) whose exact combination determined a person's temperament, with illnesses emerging when an imbalance occurred, either when the humours were said to be in excess or in deficit. They were cosmologically linked to the stars and planets, to seasonal changes, to different stages of a person's life and so on. Other theories of disease causation down the ages included the wrath of supernatural entities such as gods, configuration of the stars or miasmas.

put the last nail in the coffin of spontaneous generation by showing that it was pathogenic micro-organisms which caused damage to the silk, wine and milk industries. We owe pasteurised milk to him. He not only uncovered harmful bacteria but also harmful viruses as well – the germ theory of disease in the new "Age of Bacteriology" marked the watershed between scientific and pre-scientific or pseudo-scientific medicine. He also pioneered vaccination, developing a vaccine against rabies, a deadly disease caused by a virus in the saliva of dogs infected by it. He played the lead role introducing the concept of the Monogenic Conception of Disease which simplistically put, says: one cause/germ (bacteria), one disease, although he left it to Koch to complete the task of filling out this grand pronouncement.

Koch did it in 1876 in a paper about his findings on anthrax presented to members of the Botanical Institute in Breslau: "each disease is caused by one particular microbe – and by one alone. Only an anthrax microbe causes anthrax; only a typhoid microbe can cause typhoid fever" (Evans,1993, 20). It is the fulfilment of a long-cherished dream: "the final hope and aim of medical science is the establishment of monogenic disease entities" (Taylor, 1979, 21).[2]

This version of the Monogenic Conception of Disease as introduced by Pasteur and adopted by Koch as just set out above may be referred to as the Classical Version or the non-dogmatic version, as it serves to mark the establishment of a new paradigm of scientificity in Medical Thinking, abandoning older paradigms such as that of the Humours, the wrath of the gods and others for the Modern paradigm of micro-organisms as the relevant pathogenic variable.

However, in an attempt to clarify the new paradigm, Koch in 1890 embellished it with a set of methodological rules/guidelines to determine the cause of any particular disease which came to called either the Koch or the Henle-Koch postulates. They are:[3]

---

[2] The Monogenic Conception of Disease has also been used to pick out as causal agent, not only bacteria or viruses but also fungus (such as ringworm), parasite (such as Plasmodium which causes malaria), prion (misfolded protein which can cause Creutzfeldt-Jakob disease, a neurodegenerative disease), and genes (especially in the case of rare single-gene disorders, such as Down Syndrome). This larger conception of the Monogenic Conception of Disease which has evolved since Koch will be further explored in the next chapter, Chapter 3 when phenylketonuria attributed to a single defective gene will be critically examined.

[3] As presented by Cohen, 2017. See also Lee, 2012, Chapters 9 and 10.

1 The bacteria be present in every case of the disease and under circumstances which can account for the pathological changes and clinical course of the disease.
2 The parasite occurs in no other disease as a fortuitous and non-pathogenic parasite.
3 After being fully isolated from the body and repeatedly grown in pure culture, the parasite can induce disease anew.
4 The parasite can be re-isolated from an experimentally inoculated host.[4]

By so doing, Koch appeared to depart from the Monogenic Conception of Disease in its Classical Version (or its non-dogmatic version) and to transform it into a dogma. This is because, ironically, Koch realised that he could not carry out the Postulates as specified. For example, after he discovered the presence of the cholera bacteria in cholera sufferers in India as well as in the water tanks from which the victims had drawn their water, he injected the bacteria into animals rather than human beings for obvious ethical reasons. Yet, they remained stubbornly healthy (thereby falsifying Postulate 3). He also found that some people who carried the cholera germ also stubbornly showed no sign of the symptoms of cholera (thereby undermining Postulate 1 which as he had formulated it, which is misleadingly too wide). Strictly speaking, his findings had undermined two of his own postulates. This meant that the Monogenic Conception of Disease had already run into problems even as it was being launched to great acclaim.

However, can one salvage Postulate 1 in some way, by re-interpreting it as simply claiming that a factor/variable is a necessary condition of the disease and not as Koch maintained that it be "universal and necessary"? [5] In other words, in its absence the disease would not occur but its presence is not on its own sufficient to bring it about. If the concept of cause is to be understood in terms of necessary condition only, it would be a weak conception. A more robust conception would demand that the factor/ variable be both necessary and sufficient. However, Koch's own experiments had indicated that no single condition could function as both a necessary and sufficient condition for the occurrence of cholera, as he had also discovered that some people who were bearers of the cholera bacteria were asymptomatic – some other factor or factors must, therefore, be present before these bearers of the germ would develop the disease called cholera.

---

[4] The fourth postulate was added by later writers. See also Evans 1976 for a revised and revamped version.
[5] See Carter, 2003, 1.

However, in spite of such flaws in Koch's reasoning, he was awarded the Nobel Prize for Medicine in 1905. A caveat must straightaway be entered. These remarks are not intended to challenge the claim that Koch (together with Pasteur) founded the germ theory of disease, a radical discovery which had far-reaching consequences for human health world-wide. Instances include the following: in 1908 the germ for polio was found to be a certain virus which led eventually to the emergence of the polio vaccine in 1958; the chance discovery of penicillin by Fleming in 1928 led to the mass production of antibiotics, post-WWll, making antibiotics the standard treatment against (bacterial) infection in Clinical Medicine. Undoubtedly, many lives have been saved and will continue to be saved in spite of the resistance to antibiotics in some cases owing to the excessive use over time of such a "magic bullet". These remarks are directed at Koch's somewhat simplistic grasp of the notion of cause in medicine, especially with the wisdom of hindsight. It is to draw attention to the difference between the Monogenic Conception of Disease held in its Classical Version (not as a dogma) and when it came to be held as a dogma.

Just as some people infected with the cholera bacterium were asymptomatic, the same holds true in the case of the coronavirus SARS-CoV-2 where some infected people are also asymptomatic. This was grasped early on in the SARS-CoV-2/COVID-19 pandemic. In the UK, towards the end of January 2020 even before the first COVID-19 case was confirmed in the country, SAGE (Scientific Advisory Group for Emergencies) warned the government that asymptomatic transmission could not be ruled out. In early to mid-February 2020, a cruise ship called the Diamond Princess had quarantined its 3,711 passengers and crew when they found 712 (19.2%) infected cases, of which 410 (331/46.5%) who tested positive, nevertheless, remained asymptomatic. On 21st February 2020, *The Journal of the American Medical Association/JAMA* published a paper by Chinese scientists about asymptomatic transmission of COVID-19 (see Bai, Yao, Wei, *et al.* 2020, 1406-1407). There is also evidence for presymptomatic transmission. [6] The existence of asymptomatic as well as presymptomatic cases could mean that transmission might go undetected and hence the disease could spread more widely.

---

[6] The term "asymptomatic" should be strictly confined to those who never develop symptoms; in this sense, we can identify who are asymptomatic only in retrospect. "Presymptomatic" should be reserved for those people who show no symptoms when they get a positive test result but who eventually develop the symptoms. In the case of SARS-CoV-2, one must wait approximately 14 days before determining whether symptoms have developed. For evidence of presymptomatic transmission, see: Accessed January 25, 2023. https://pubmed.ncbi.nlm.nih.gov/32767657/ .

In other words, the existence of asymptomatic cases should alert medical scientists to the plausible criticism that the model of causation in infectious disease could not be that endorsed by the Monogenic Conception of Disease (held as dogma) as it is too simplistic. The issue about what model of causation could be said to be more adequate is mentioned now but not pursued as its detailed exploration will take place in later chapters (from Chapter 5 onwards). Instead, one focusses, here, on testing the conception against the discovery of another pathogen, this time a bacterium, in the case of *Helicobacter pylori* by Barry Marshall (physician) and Robert Warren (pathologist) in 2005 as the cause of peptic ulcer disease, a discovery which overturned the extant explanation in terms of stress, spicy foods and/or too much acid in the stomach. In this context, the discovery amounts to the Classical Version of the Monogenic Conception of Disease.

However, to go beyond the enunciation of it as the Classical Version could be misleading and runs into the danger of adhering to the Monogenic Conception of Disease as dogma. Let us pose the question: Is *H. pylori* a sufficient condition of peptic ulcer? To say, that it is, entails that every person (ascertained by the usual means such as through endoscopy) who has *H. pylori* in the stomach would have the disease called peptic ulcer disease whose symptoms include the following: belching, feeling pain, sick, vomiting, sometimes bleeding via vomiting blood or passing blood in bowel movements. What does medical data in fact show? It shows that 90% of people known to have *H. pylori* infection do not develop gastritis or peptic ulcers. Only 10% do. As a matter of fact, roughly 80% of the world's population harbours *H. pylori* of which only 10% have the disease. In other words, large numbers are asymptomatic. To say that the factor X (the cause) is a sufficient condition for Y (the effect) is to say that the occurrence of X guarantees the occurrence of Y. However, we have just shown that the presence of X (*H. pylori*) fails invariably to guarantee Y (the effect/peptic ulcer disease).

If not a sufficient condition, is it, then, a necessary condition? It appears not. First, let us distinguish between the sufferers in two very different contexts: (a) 90% of peptic ulcer disease in the world are caused by *H. pylori* infection – sufferers in developing countries are, in the main, caused by such infection; (b) however, this leaves 10% of sufferers, living primarily in the developed world whose disease is not caused by *H. pylori* infection. Their ulcers are caused by excessive use of NSAIDs (non-steroidal anti-inflammatory drugs such as aspirin, ibuprofen, naproxen sodium). About 30 per cent of regular NSAID users have one or more ulcers. It follows that the peptic ulcer disease can occur even in the absence of the putative cause, *H. pylori*.

If above criticism is plausible, that *H. pylori* is neither a necessary nor a sufficient condition of peptic ulcer disease, then the Monogenic Conception of Disease is severely undermined, not only more than a hundred years ago when Koch singled out the cholera bacterium, as the cause of cholera but also about two decades ago when adherence to the Monogenic Conception of Disease (held beyond the Classical Version) seems to have failed yet again to obtain in the causal relation between peptic ulcer disease and *H. Pylori.*

Mackie, 1974, exploring the notion of cause in the explanatory/ scientific context argues that no factor should be singled out as "the cause" as each of several relevant factors identified, taken on its own, is neither necessary nor sufficient, although each is a necessary component of this particular complex. In other words, all identified factors form a complex set of "inus conditions". For instance, should we wish to explain why a person exposed to SARS-CoV-2 succumbs to COVID-19, we may find a set of relevant conditions such as the person's age, health-status (any co-morbidities), past illnesses (which may have lingering effects), place and kind of employment, lifestyle characteristics such as diet, and so forth. Of course, in any one case of infection, not all of these conditions would obtain but it is certainly the case as indicated by the data that any one case of infection would involve one or more of such factors apart from exposure to and infection by SARS-CoV-2. According to Mackie, "inus" stands for "an insufficient but necessary part of an unnecessary but sufficient complex".

Take this example from Wulff 1984, 169-177 to illustrate what could be meant by "inus conditions". A male patient presents himself with a stiff neck and a high temperature. The doctors put him through certain diagnostic tests from the results of which, they diagnosed meningitis as his spinal fluid contained pneumococci. His records showed that he had no spleen as it had been removed [7] following an accident earlier on in his life and that he had not been vaccinated against pneumococcal infections. What then is "the cause" of his meningitis should we follow the Monogenic Conception of Disease (beyond its Classical Version)? The removal of the spleen? or the failure to vaccinate him against pneumococcal infections following the splenectomy? Or is it the pneumococci in his spinal fluid? Strictly speaking, adherence to the Monogenic Conception of Disease permits one in logic to opt for one of the three mentioned factors, namely, the pneumococci in the patient's spinal fluid. The important point to grasp is that each of these three conditions, on its own, is neither necessary nor sufficient for the patient's

[7] People whose spleen has been removed are prone to an increased incidence of pneumococcal infections as well as to other sorts of infection such as sepsis.

suffering from meningitis. All three factors in combination cause the meningitis – this complex set of relevant factors constituted a set of "inus conditions" of the patient's meningitis. To labour the point, each of the said variables occurring in the set of "inus conditions", on its own, is neither a necessary nor a sufficient condition of the meningitis diagnosed in the patient.

The Henle-Koch postulates were formulated in the 1890s and a lot of water has passed under the bridge of what today we call biomedicine. As Cohen 2017 puts it:

> Koch's postulates were invaluable at the time they were developed and remain largely valid for a relatively small number of defined circumstances in which bacteria can be precisely tied to the cause of a particular clinical syndrome. But in a world in which virus cause cancer and noncultivable bacteria can be demonstrated by molecular probes, Koch's postulates are no longer fit for purpose. … Their main purpose now is to provide a framework to ensure that scientific rigor is applied when proposing an organism as the cause of a disease – exactly as Koch intended when he first conceived them.

Stewart 1968 (already mentioned in the last chapter) has put the point well – that the conception has become a dogma. He wrote:

> The germ theory of disease – infectious disease is generally caused by transmission of an organism from one host to another – is a gross oversimplification. It accords with the basic facts that infection without an organism is impossible and that transmissible organisms can cause disease; but it does not explain the exceptions and anomalies. The germ theory has become a dogma because it neglects the many other factors which have a part to play in deciding whether the host/germ/ environment complex is to lead to infection. Among these are susceptibility, generic constitution, behaviour, and socioeconomic determinants. (*The Lancet*, May 18, 1968, 1077).

Another way of making roughly the same point is to say that a model of causality to be adequate to explain any disease/illness, but especially in an epidemic or pandemic such as COVID-19 must include both necessary and sufficient conditions. This is to remind the lay person that citing SARS-CoV-2 as the cause of COVID-19 is only to cite a necessary condition and not both its necessary and sufficient conditions.[8] However, sometimes, the medical

---

[8] For readers who are not over-familiar with causal discourse, an example to illustrate the distinction between necessary and sufficient conditions may be

professionals forget to say explicitly that when they say that the coronavirus is "the cause" of COVID-19, they are really talking about the understanding of or referring to cause only as necessary condition, not as both necessary and sufficient conditions. Examples may be found in the recent literature about the epidemic or pandemic of this oversight, some of which are cited below:

WHO. (April 2023). [9] Overview: "Coronavirus disease (COVID-19) is an infectious disease caused by the SARS-CoV-2 virus".
CDC (USA): COVID-19. (Updated Nov. 4, 2021). [10] "COVID-19 is caused by a virus called SARS-CoV-2".

Nature: nature reviews microbiology. 19, 141-154 (2021). (06 October 2020).[11] "At the end of 2019, a novel coronavirus designated as SARS-CoV-2 emerged in the city of Wuhan, China, and caused an outbreak of unusual viral pneumonia"; "…the causative agent of this emerging disease is a betacoronavirus that had never been seen before".

Johns Hopkins Medicine. (Updated July 29, 2022). [12] "A coronavirus identified in 2019, SARS-CoV-2, has caused a pandemic of respiratory illness, called COVID-19." "COVID-19 is the disease caused by SARS-CoV-2, the coronavirus that emerged in December 2019."

---

appropriately invoked here. Take a fire. For a fire to take place, oxygen must be present in the air. This is to say that oxygen is a necessary condition of the occurrence of a fire – in the absence of oxygen, no fire can take place. However, the presence of oxygen in the atmosphere is not sufficient to bring about a fire – other conditions must also exist at the same time which are sufficient to generate fire as the outcome, such as the presence of inflammable material (say a wooden hut containing wood shavings, a stroke of lightening hitting the shed or some vandal passing by who throws his lighted cigarette onto the wood shavings. The oxygen (a necessary condition) plus the wooden hut containing the wood shavings plus the carelessly abandoned cigarette (the sufficient conditions) together would or could account for the fire as the causal outcome.

[9] "Coronavirus disease (COVID-19)". Accessed April 4, 2023, https://www. who. int/health-topics/coronavirus#tab=tab_1 .

[10] "Basics of COVID-19". Accessed April 4, 2023. https://www.cdc.gov /coronavirus/ 2019-ncov/your-health/about-covid-19/basics-covid-19.html .

[11] "Characteristics of SARS-CoV-2 and COVID-19" (by Ben Hu, Hua Gao, Peng Zhou & Zheng-Li Shi). (uploaded on 06/10/2020). Accessed April 4, 2023. https://www.nature.com/articles/s41579-020-00459-7 .

[12] "What Is Coronavirus?" Accessed April 4, 2023.
https://www. hopkinsmedicine.org/health/conditions-and-diseases/coronavirus .

Conclusion

1. To say simplistically that "the cause" of COVID-19 is the coronavirus, SARS-CoV-2 may be misleading, especially to the lay person, as it masks the complexity of the causal scene. It is inappropriate to pose the What question and then to answer it in terms of the coronavirus.
2. In part, the "instinct" to pronounce in such a simplistic manner may be traced to the highly prestigious conception of disease called the Monogenic Conception of Disease which is considered to have ushered in the modern age of scientific medicine in Clinical Medicine, with Pasteur and Koch as the giants leading the field. This prestigious conception may be called the Classical Version and may be lauded as the non-dogmatic version as it can be understood to articulate a new paradigm of scientificity in Medical Thinking for the Modern Age which in the case of infectious diseases explain disease/illness in terms of pathogenic micro-organisms which have invaded the patient's body.
3. However, subjecting Koch's postulates (sometimes also called the Henle-Koch postulates) to critical scrutiny by testing them against available medical data in the SARS-CoV-2/COVID-19 context shows that Postulate 1, in particular, which is key to the Monogenic Conception of Disease (held as dogma) is methodologically flawed.
4. Re-testing them but this time using the case of peptic ulcer disease and *H. pylori* as the causative agent, a hundred or more years after Koch, also throws up the same flaws in the Monogenic Conception of Disease.
5. The logic of that conception of disease which has since its appearance taken on the status of a dogma (until of late, say, post 1968) is so restrictive that it cannot cope with what Mackie called "inus conditions", a set of relevant factors which together in combination generates the disease/illness in question, although each of these relevant conditions, on its own, separate from the others, is neither necessary nor sufficient for the occurrence of the disease/illness.
6. The reader should always bear in mind that any adequate model of causality should include both the necessary and the sufficient conditions for the generation of a disease/illness, including a highly infectious one such as COVID-19 in an epidemic or pandemic. To say that SARS-CoV-2 is "the cause" of COVID-19 is just to say that it is a necessary condition for the generation of the disease and not that it is both necessary and sufficient. The set of necessary and sufficient conditions include many other factors such as "susceptibility, generic constitution, behaviour, and socioeconomic determinants" as aptly observed by Stewart 1968.

7 One ought to point out an ironical turn of events in Marshall's and Warren's discovery of the *H. pylori* as the cause of peptic ulcer disease. They spent up to twenty years to get the thesis first accepted and then to obtain the Nobel Prize in Medicine in 2005. This was because the medical community, for a considerable period of time, could not accept that bacteria could live and survive under acidic conditions in the stomach of a patient. So, they stuck to the view current at the time, that peptic ulcers were caused by stress and other lifestyle factors, not by a micro-organism. Marshall and Warren had difficulty getting medical journals, such as *The Lancet* from accepting their submission. Finally, in desperation, Marshall resorted to swallowing the pathogenic bacteria after first making sure that he was free from peptic ulcer disease at the beginning of the experiment, and that he became infected with it through the experiment. (See *The Lancet* 2005.) In other words, Marshall invoked (though not consciously) Collingwood's understanding of cause via manipulation and control (see Chapter 5). In this way, Marshall carried out Koch's Postulate 3. Marshall's heroic act paid off, as he was successful in pulling off the experiment on himself. He was lucky, but he need not have been. Remember Koch's experiment with cholera on animals? Those animals remained steadfastly asymptomatic. In any case, Marshall could, in principle, belong to that 90% of people in the world known to have *H. pylori* infection but who do not develop gastritis or peptic ulcers. Only 10% do. Statistics show that 80% of the world's population harbour *H. pylori* of which only 10% have the disease. In other words, large numbers are asymptomatic. His experiment of a single participant, that is himself, in any case, is not compatible with the normal guidelines for scientificity in conducting experiments. In other words, methodologically, Marshall was not standing on firm ground.

CHAPTER 3

WHO MANIFESTS A DISEASE? A CUT-AND-DRY MATTER?

This chapter continues the critique of the Monogenic Conception of Disease held as dogma by scrutinising in some detail the question: **W**ho manifests a disease/illness? Chapter 2 has examined the related **W**hat question and found the conception wanting when applied in the context of either a pathogenic virus (SARS-CoV-2 in the case of COVID-19) or a pathogenic bacterium (*H. pylori* in the case of peptic ulcer disease). These two cases involve infectious diseases. However, the Monogenic Conception of Disease claims a wider remit than viral and bacterial infection. In its widest understanding, it simply reads: one pathogenic cause, one effect. Pathogenic viruses and bacteria fit nicely into this formula which, however, is not limited to them only. For instance, defective genes could count as a pathogenic factor for disease-generation. Hence, this chapter focuses on phenylketonuria, a disease attributed to a defective gene, to see if the same criticism about the Monogenic Conception of Disease also obtains in this context, namely, that it cannot do justice to all the relevant data which constitute the complexity of disease-generation. This **W**ho question, like the **W**hat question, can only be adequately addressed by abandoning that conception of disease (held as dogma) and opting for a multifactorial model of relationships between two and/or more relevant variables, namely, the bi-directional, multifactorial mode of causation/BMC and not the unidirectional, monofactorial mode of causation/UMC.

Who is the Individual Person with the Disease?

Chapter 2 has already drawn attention to an important aspect of infection in an epidemic/pandemic, namely, that not all those who have been exposed to the germ in question and become infected by it will automatically exhibit symptoms of the disease. The data in the case of SARS-CoV-2/COVID-19 (published in May 2021) appear to show that at least one third of infected cases are asymptomatic.[1] However, asymptomatic infection occurs not only with infection from a virus but also from pathogenic bacteria, such as *H. pylori* which is said to be "the cause" of peptic ulcer disease. Just to remind the reader, it turns out that although 80% of the world's population are bearers of *H. pylori* only 10% of them develop peptic ulcer disease. [2] This observation does not simply serve to undermine the validity of the Monogenic Conception of Disease (held as dogma) but is also a compelling signal for much needed research and investigation why this is so. No-body to date would and could claim to know as much as is desired, but a fair number of medical scientists may be prepared to argue that they must look beyond the simplistic Reductionist temptation offered by genetics (in its triumphalist phase following the discovery of the double helix structure of the DNA molecule by Crick and Watson in 1953) to answer the question – see Noble, 2006.

That early triumphalism was finally knocked on its head when the Human Genome Project, upon its completion, made known its findings in 2003. Contrary to expectation, the number of genes uncovered were relatively few, only probably about 20,500 genes when estimates had ranged from 50,000 to as many as 140,000. Science had to do some serious re-thinking. That is why Noble confessed that although he had spent the greater part of his career doing Reductionist science, he felt the need to change tack, to abandon Reductionism and to opt for a "systems"/Wholist approach. [3]

Although no rational person would doubt that genetic endowment plays a role in the individual's appearance and behaviour, no well-informed

---

[1] See Oran and Topol 2021; Ma, Liu, Liu, *et al.* 2021 for systematic reviews of available data.

[2] Peptic ulcer disease is not considered to be a pandemic minimally for three reasons: (a) infection though extensive and widespread throughout the globe is not considered to be alarming as only a minority of the infected shows symptoms of the disease; (b) those infected live mainly in the developing economies and (c) given that the mode of transmission of peptic ulcer disease does not affect people in the developed economies, there is little or no incentive to do anything about the matter. In contrast, SARS-CoV-2 is alarming as given its mode of transmission, developed economies could readily fall prey to it as, indeed, they have and continue to do so (in late August 2022, at the time of writing this chapter), grappling with BA.4 and BA.5 which are variants of the original Omicron virus, with the number of cases world-wide standing at just below 600 million and deaths world-wide at roughly 6 and a half million – see some figures, dated 10/07/2022, in Table 4.1 in chapter which follows, Chapter 4.

[3] See Chapter 1 for a clarification about the use of the terms "Wholist" and "Wholism". See Chapter 7 which explores Wholism via the concept of ecosystem-nesting.

person today would hold the view that the genotype determines the phenotype. We now know enough about the science of genetics to know that the genes in the human genome are themselves complexly related. See Figure 3.1 below:

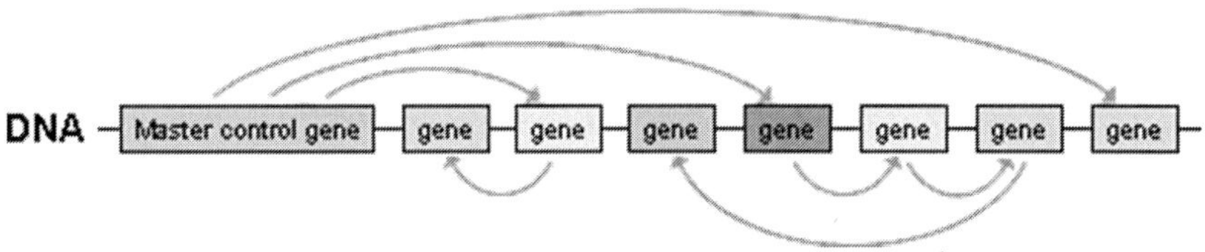

Figure 3.1. Complex relationships between genes [4]

Developmental biology invokes the concept of a master gene, that is, a single gene whose expression constitutes the appropriate conditions for activating many other genes in a co-ordinated manner, ultimately leading to a specific tissue or organ being developed. Pax-6 is said to be such a gene which triggers development of the eye. However, what needs emphasising is that development of any cell, tissue, organ, or whole organism depends on more than the existence of genes, as the environment, both internal and external plays a critical role in human biology in particular and in biology in general. See Figure 3.2 below:

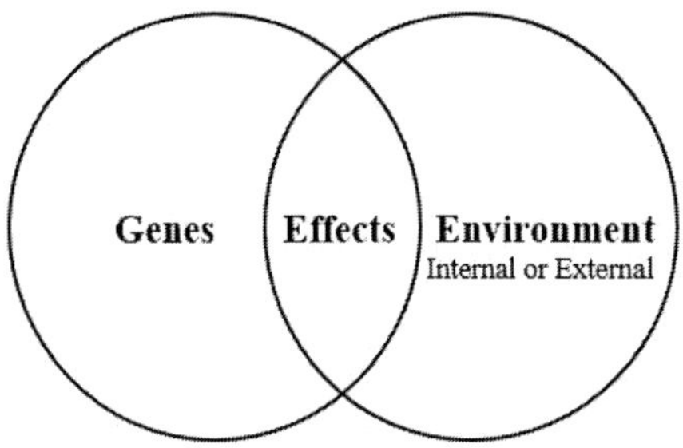

Figure 3.2 Genes interacting with environmental factors, internal and/or external.

Genes, we know, are embedded in cells; we also know that the internal as well as the external environment of a cell can affect which genes are "turned on", so to speak. For instance, hormones can "tell" a cell to activate

[4] Accessed and downloaded July 14, 2022.
https://evolution.berkeley.edu/ evo library/images/evo/control_gene.gif.

a specific gene (internal environmental factor). [5] Experimental data exist which confirm that outside temperature can affect the expression of the gene controlling the colour of fur in rabbits (external environmental factor). An ice pack was strapped to the back of a rabbit with white body fur. At the end of the experiment, when the ice pack was removed, one would find that the rabbit had a patch of much darker fur on its back in exactly the place where the ice pack was – see "Role of Environmental Factors in Gene Expression" 2012.

To clarify further what Figure 3.2 above means, take the case of the disease called phenylketonuria. Although disorders may involve single faulty genes, it does not mean that the disease would necessarily manifest itself. Phenylketonuria is one such instance. [6] In many countries, infants when born are tested to see if they have inherited this condition and in the rare cases where they have, their parents are immediately advised to put the child on a diet (probably lasting a lifetime) to avoid foods which are rich in phenylalanine, as the inherited defective gene means that the body cannot make an enzyme called phenylalanine hydroxylase (PAH), an enzyme necessary for converting the amino acid phenylalanine into other substances the body needs. Most forms of phenylketonuria are caused by mutations in the PAH gene on chromosome 12q23.2. The defective PAH gene then leads to the accumulation of the amino acid in the blood, causing a whole range of conditions (intellectual disability, delayed development, behavioural and social problems, psychiatric disorders and so forth), from mild to severe. In other words, the disease will manifest itself or the gene would only be "activated"/expressed in the presence of certain adverse environmental factors.

The external environment of the individual would naturally include other people and their behaviour/attitude, whether these others are aware of the person's dietary needs or are conscientious in implementing such a dietary regime or helping them to implement such a regime. If the external environment is not hospital to meeting the person's dietary needs, they would likely ingest foods rich in phenylalanine which then become part of their internal environment, wreaking havoc upon it.

The above complex interacting relationships are hardly amenable to the Monogenic Conception of Disease model of disease (held as dogma) and its implied UMC; rather they appear to go hand in hand with what may be

---

[5] See Ing 2005 for a review of the literature on how steroid hormones regulate gene expression.

[6] PKU is what is called an autosomal recessive metabolic genetic disorder. As such it requires two PKU alleles (one from each parent) to be present in individuals before they would experience symptoms of the disease.

called multifactorial inheritance (or polygenic) disorders, such as heart disease, diabetes, obesity and most cancers. These are caused by a combination of small inherited variations in genes but acting in conjunction with certain adverse environmental factors (namely, Mackie's "inus conditions").

Phenylketonuria is a clear instance of what may be called synergism at work. The faulty gene on its own may not produce the brain damage; neither does a normal diet relatively high in phenylalanine (in the absence of the faulty gene). Each of the factors cited, on its own, does not bring about brain damage. Yet when the factors happen to combine, then and only then, does brain damage occur. The brain damage is the synergistic effect of all these causally relevant factors. Under synergism, the total effect is more than or is different from the sum of the effects of each of these factors when measured separately on its own. Synergism in certain contexts could lead even to death. Such as taking sleeping pills and alcohol, if an individual were to swallow more than the number of sleeping pills prescribed for their condition, this on its own would not necessarily kill the person, although they may cause some very unpleasant effects. Similarly, if the person were to drink half a bottle of whisky on its own, a very nasty hangover the next day would ensue. However, should the individual swallow the pills at the same time as consuming the alcohol, then death could, and would ensue in certain instances, if the attempt combining both was not discovered in time by others.

The case of phenylketonuria handily illustrates the complex relationship between the gene/host relationship when that relationship operates within a larger environment which itself can be broken up into three sub-environments, namely, the physical, the social as well as the chemical and biological – see the version here (Figure 3.3 below) of what is found in Bhopal, 2008, 135. The host/person possesses the gene defect which leads to an enzyme deficiency which, in turn, may lead to brain damage. The host/person operates within a larger (physical-social) environment which includes facilities for early diagnosis, as early diagnosis backed up by dietary control could help prevent/control the manifestation of the disease. The host/person also operates within a specific social environment which includes active support to make it possible to sustain on a long-term basis the special dietary regimen, if prevention/control were to be effective. Such special diet, if conscientiously sustained, would mean that the host's chemical and biological environment would be such that the disease would not manifest itself in the lifetime of the host. This enlarged wheel model of causal complexity shows very clearly that it would be distorting to regard phenylketonuria simplistically as a genetic disease in which its "cause" is a gene defect *tout court*. Phenylketonuria is also an environmental disease.

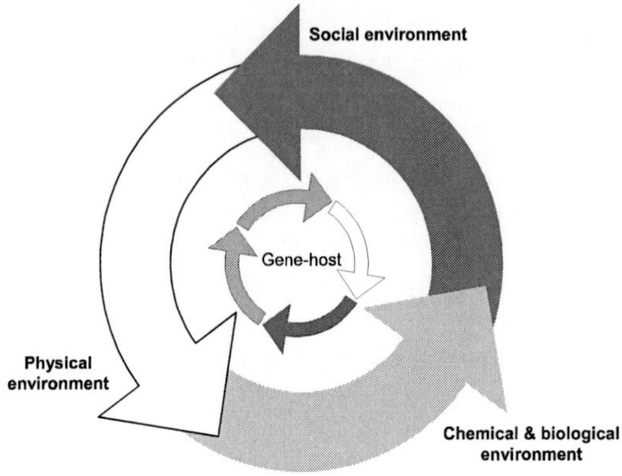

Figure 3.3 Three external environments acting upon the Gene-host with its own internally complex interactions in generating phenylketonuria.

In other words, whether the outcome is related to a defective gene as in the case of phenylketonuria or to pathogenic bacteria, *H. pylori* as in peptic ulcer disease, or to a virus, SARS-CoV-2 as in COVID-19, environmental (physical and social) factors play a critical role in disease-generation/illness when they act in tandem with a gene/bacteria/virus. From this, one may plausibly conclude that diseases do not conform to the Monogenic Conception of Disease model of disease-generation (held simplistically and as dogma) and its implied UMC.

Conclusion

1 This chapter subjects the Monogenic Conception of Disease-UMC to test by confronting it with data from yet another context of disease-generation, the case of phenylketonuria where a defective gene is said to play the definitive role and, hence, has been singled out as "the cause" of the disease called phenylketonuria.
2 However, a critical examination shows that the conclusion of the Monogenic Conception of Disease in this context (held simplistically and as dogma) is not justified. Phenylketonuria, just like peptic ulcer disease and COVID-19, does not conform to the Monogenic Conception of Disease account of disease-generation (held as dogma).
3 All three diseases would not, and could not be generated except when the problematic item (in phenylketonuria it is the PAH gene, in peptic ulcer disease, it is the pathogenic bacteria, *H. pylori* and in COVID-19,

it is the pathogenic virus [7] SARS-CoV-2) acts in combination with a set of adverse environmental (internal and external) circumstances which lead to the generation of the disease in question.

4 The **Who** question cannot be answered by simply saying: The person manifesting the disease is the person who has the defective gene (or the pathogenic bacteria or the pathogenic virus).

5 In other words, disease-generation factors are not only items studied in a pathology lab, Clinical Medicine includes environmental factors which fall more readily into the other domain of biomedicine, that of Epidemiology.

Advance in biomedicine regarding diagnosis and treatment comes about through the fruitful co-operation between Clinical Medicine and Epidemiology. Epidemiology plays a role equal in importance to that of Clinical Medicine; it need not and should not be stigmatised with the label of being inferior to its counterpart, Clinical Medicine.

[7] Note that just as not all bacteria are pathogenic from the point of view of human health, not all viruses are pathogenic. Genomic studies of human samples from healthy people have increasingly found evidence of unrecognised viruses in intestines, lungs, skin and blood, many of which appear to be harmless. Some of these symbiotic viruses can provide protection against other pathogenic viruses. For instance, a virus of the same family as the hepatitis C virus, the Zika virus and the dengue virus is reported as actually capable of reducing the symptoms of HIV infection. See Mathew 2019; The Teller Report 2020.

CHAPTER 4

SPATIAL-TEMPORAL ASPECTS OF DISEASE-GENERATION: THE WHERE AND WHEN QUESTIONS

This chapter adopts a slightly different strategy as it tests the Monogenic Conception of Disease yet again, but this time in the context of two questions, the **W**here and the **W**hen questions. The former question addresses the spatial aspect while the latter, the temporal. Together, they bring to the foreground the relevance of Epidemiology to the understanding of disease-generation and disease-transmission of a pathogenic virus, such as SARS-CoV-2. At the same time, their exploration also demonstrates the contribution of Clinical Medicine to understanding the transmission of COVID-19 as an infectious disease. In other words, it is only through the joint effort of Clinical Medicine and Epidemiology that we can hope to get on top of the disease to control it. It will also link the **W**here and **W**hen questions with the **W**ho question via the group of the elderly in order to demonstrate the interrelated nature of all three in disease-generation.

The SARS-CoV-2 Virus: Where and When is an Individual Likely to Meet It?

To answer this question, as already observed, one needs the help of Clinical Medicine. Towards the end of 2019, Wuhan, China reported cases of a new severe acute respiratory syndrome. This puzzled the medical community world-wide, in spite of the fact that it had experience in dealing with an outbreak of SARS (severe acute respiratory syndrome) in China in 2002-2003 as well as of MERS (Middle East respiratory syndrome) in 2012. However, although coronaviruses are implicated in all three, they are also different. For instance, the new acute respiratory distress syndrome consists of some pathogenetic, epidemiological and clinical features which were not completely understood at the time of their emergence. Very soon, the medical world recovered from the jolt and pulled resources together to get on top of the phenomenon. Medical scientists in China established that the first 27 documented hospitalised cases were epidemiologically traced to Huanan wholesale seafood market, a wet market in Wuhan city.[1] In retrospect, it was also established that the first known cases dated back to the 8 December 2019. On 31 December, China notified the World Health Organisation/WHO of such an outbreak, keeping themselves and the scientific community world-wide informed of the results of its medical investigation, including the first genome sequence of the virus on 10 January 2020, followed by more completed genome sequences on 12 January 2020. Their work also established that there was clear evidence of human-to-human transmission of the new virus. In the light of such information, the WHO on 30 January 2020 declared the novel outbreak a public health emergency of international concern ("PHEIC") and on 11 March 2020, used the common term "pandemic".[2] On 11 February 2020,

---

[1] In retrospect, this hypothesis turns out not to be as strong as it was at first sight thought to be, although it may not be wise to discard it altogether. This, at least, is the opinion of Jeffrey Sachs, lead author of the *Lancet* Commission on COVID-19. On 19 May 2022, he urged a serious, transparent investigation by the scientific community of the two contending hypotheses of the origin of SARS-CoV-2, namely the zoonotic and lab-leak – see Harrison and Sachs 2022. However, around mid-March 2023, new data emerged which appear to support the zoonotic hypothesis, mentioning the racoon dog as a possible agent of transmission. See Mueller 2023. See also the latest release of researchers at the Chinese Disease Control and Prevention of the swabs collected at the market – "COVID-origins data from Wuhan market published: what scientists think" (05 April 2023); "China must share data on COVID-19's origins 'immediately,' WHO scientist demands" (06/04/2023).

The latest (the third study in two months) analysis of genomic data from the Wuhan market swabs (*Nature Briefing* May 4, 2023) now maintains that the samples collected in the early weeks of the pandemic are "of limited value for pinpointing which animal species – if any, infected people at the market…" However, virologists still consider these analyses of scientific worth as they confirm that specific wild animals which could have been infected with SARS-CoV-2 (such as the bamboo rat, the racoon dog) were at the market before its closure. Furthermore, the virologist George Gao at the China CDC (and lead author of the *Nature* study) is reported as saying: "We do not have anything of the earlier sequencing data from China CDC that have not been shared with the world. The origin of the virus is a scientific question and remains elusive." (See also Bloom 2023; *The Intercept* 2023).

[2] However, the term "pandemic" is considered to be legally and operationally distinct from PHEIC, although it is often used interchangeably with it in the context of the COVID-19 outbreak. The WHO might have first called the COVID-19 phenomenon a pandemic in March 2020; however, a spokesperson of the WHO, nearly three years later in early 2023 clarified that this should not be read to mean

the International Committee on Taxonomy of Viruses named the novel coronavirus "SARS-CoV-2" and the WHO named the disease "COVID-19".

The medical scientists initially were none too clear about the exact manner in which SARS-CoV-2 spread itself. At an earlier stage, they thought that it used the (large) droplet route, called fomite transmission, the same route as taken by the influenza virus. It led them to recommend strategies such as constant cleaning of surfaces with disinfectants and hands with sanitisers as well as frequent hand-washing with soap. In the UK, the then Prime Minster, Boris Johnson, even suggested that people should sing the popular ditty "Happy Birthday" as a ready marker of how long the hand-washing should last to be effective. Some people became so obsessed with disinfecting and washing that they started even to disinfect the packaging of groceries. In some cases, too much cleaning and using disinfectants even caused adverse acute and chronic health problems. A good deal of resources were devoted to the task of avoiding infection, presenting a problem to some small businesses who found it hard to bear the additional outlay.

However, in the light of fuller investigation, the medical experts downplayed fomite transmission and instead, focussed on small droplet and aerosol transmission, as the primary mode. [3] When people who have been infected by SARS-CoV-2 speak, cough, sneeze and so forth, they transmit particles of the virus via droplets and aerosols, with the larger droplets falling on certain surfaces (fomites). These infected surfaces may then be transferred to a person who happened to touch them. In turn, such a person could transmit to another via (smaller) droplets and aerosols which could subsequently enter the mucous membranes of a susceptible host. When the lungs expel droplets, they vary in size from very large particles which quickly fall to the ground because of gravity within a distance of 2 m or 6 ft, to the vast majority which are smaller that stay aloft for between 30 minutes and several hours and can travel beyond 2 m or 6 ft. [4]

---

that the agency had declared a pandemic, as it does not possess the mandate or power to declare the start or end of a pandemic. The spokesperson emphasised that the term "pandemic" merely "characterized the situation". See Adam 2023, 201-202.

On May 5, 2023, the WHO announced that it was ending the PHEIC it declared more than three years ago on 30 January 2020, although WHO officials and other experts warned that the lifting of the emergency should not be read as a signal that the pandemic is over. Dr Maria Van Kerkhove, the WHO top expert on COVID-19 is quoted as saying: "The emergency phase is over, but Covid is not" (*The New York Times* 2023 (May 5).

[3] See Chen (Tina) 2021.

[4] Chapter 8 will take up this issue again in the context of mask-wearing.

Given such data from virological investigation (lab science), Epidemiologists began to draw up measures to reduce the hazards of airborne transmission and avoid the risk of superspreader events. The "rules of engagement" include: keeping physical and social distancing measures (the 2 m or 6 ft rule), avoiding large crowds (such as sporting events), holding meetings in the outdoors as much as possible, and if indoor ones are to be held, then ensure adequate efficient ventilation, mask-wearing, physical distancing and so forth. [5]

China adopted the full suite of non-pharmaceutical, typically, epidemiological measures from testing/tracing/tracking importantly linked with the goal of isolating infected individuals from the rest of the population as well as physical/social distancing, mask wearing and lockdown. The results of testing were quick with people being told to stay in the clinic in which the testing was conducted. If they tested positive, they would stay in designated medical facilities until they were found virus-free as indicated by two consecutive PCR (polymerase chain reaction) tests.[6] Individuals who had come in contact with infectious people were asked to self-isolate at home for two weeks. The above-mentioned strategies proved so effective that they succeeded in minimising the length and severity of the lockdowns in most of the country (in Shanghai, its lockdown lasted just a little over three weeks with most people being free to leave their homes) [7] and even cut down transmission to very close to zero quickly. (See Falush 2020.)

According to one estimate, in the *British Medical Journal* 2021 (February 11), the data for China were as follows: 3870 deaths out of a total of 4600 identified with COVID-19; the total amount of identified infected cases country-wise were 80,000 of which Wuhan registered 50,000. According to The Johns Hopkins University CSSE COVID-19 Data as reported by Our World in Data, the cumulative confirmed figures for death

---

[5] See Sachs, Horton, Bagenal, Amor, Caman and Lafortune. 2020. *The Lancet* COVID-19 Commission.

[6] There are two types of test, the PCR and the RAT (rapid antigen test). The RAT may be self-tested and its results known almost instantaneously. The PCR test is regarded as the gold standard as it is accurate and reliable.

[7] China as a country implemented lockdown on 23 January 2020 and lifted it officially on 8 April 2020. This national lockdown lasted about two and a half months.

On the subject whether lockdown is an effective non-pharmaceutical strategy to pursue in the context of an epidemic/pandemic such as the SARS-CoV-2/COVID-19 outbreak, see "Did the COVID-19 lockdowns work? Here's what we know two years on" 2022. Its conclusion is that lockdown is effective.

were: 4,632 on 18 April 2020, and 5,226 on 7 July 2022. Here is another set of revealing figures also from Our World in Data (as of 22 March 2022).

	Cases	Deaths
USA	79.7 M (+ 25,459)	972K (+1,002)
India	43 M (+ 1,778)	517K (+ 62)
China (mainland)	137K (+ 4,569)	4,638
Hong Kong	1.08 M (+ 13,166) Or c 1,270,000[b]	6,364 (+ 245) Or c 9,400[b]

Table 4.1 Identified COVID-19 Cases and Fatalities in Four Different Locations World-wide.[8] Numbers marked with [b] are those taken from Worldometer, updated on 10/07/2022.

The figures speak for themselves.[9] Bear in mind the following points: Only India and China are comparable in terms of their population size – according to the UN records (May 2021) China was said to have an estimated population of 1.43 billion and India 1.37 billion. The US in 2021 had c 330 million, which is roughly equivalent to a fourth of China's and India's respective figures. What is even more staggering is the dramatic difference between Hong Kong and China (mainland) – Hong Kong had in 2021 just over seven and a half million people, yet its raw COVID-19 death figure was higher than that of China by roughly a third, even using the Our World in Data figures rather than those provided by Worldometer.[10] (However, let the reader be immediately reminded of the fact that these figures cited in Table 4.1 holds true especially in the case of China till say end of November 2022. The Chinese government in Beijing changed its mind in December 2022, overturning its zero-COVID-19 policy. Chapter 8 will be assessing its new policy between December 2022 and April 2023.)

---

[8] Although Hong Kong is not a sovereign state but part of China, yet under the official agreement that China recognises Hong Kong's autonomy under the "one country two systems" rule, it is legitimate in this context to include the island in the table.

[9] This is not the place to address fully the controversy surrounding the issue whether it makes sense to compare countries when they differ so much in terms of numbers alone as well as other characteristics, such as literacy rate, poverty rate, whether health services are readily available/accessible to those who require them, the level of infra-structural facilities in the community/society and so forth.

[10] In March 2022, there were nearly 900 confirmed infections per 100,000 Hong Kong citizens, surpassing the record of 500 cases per 100,000 people in January 2022 held by New York.

The dire situation in Hong Kong gives us a clue about the need to link the two **W**hen and **W**here questions with the earlier **W**ho question. Experts have tried to explain Hong Kong's extraordinary position in the world in its various spikes in terms of the following factors: its population density living in cramped spaces, especially in public housing estates, its low rates of prior infection, low vaccination rates among the elderly people, an overwhelmed healthcare system, less efficient vaccines (Sinovac) against the Omicron variants than say, Pfizer-BionTech vaccines. Those most badly affected were/are in fact the elderly. Amongst the vaccinated, the figure is a mere 37% among those aged 80 and above, compared with 81% of those aged 12 and above. (See Hutton 2022.) People over 65 accounted for 16% of the U.S. population but according to the Centre for Disease Control and Prevention/CDC, out of more than 114,000 COVID-19 associated deaths between May and August 2020, 78% of those who died were aged 65 and older (CDC, USA 2021). In India those over 60 years of age constituted just 19% of coronavirus patients in India but accounted for 63% of the deaths – see Dey 2020. [11]

We know that in general the elderly are frailer in health than younger groups. Some of its members may have co-morbidities such as diabetes, renal insufficiency, arthritis and may suffer from immunosenescence, not to mention dementia – all these combine to make them more prone to infections. Some of them because of these conditions may no longer live independently and reside in care/nursing homes which, in turn, may expose them to further risk of infection. A disturbing incidence illustrating the last point occurred in England (March-June 2020) when the government in panic-mode ordered the National Health Services/NHS hospitals to discharge 25,000 patients into care homes without any proper provision in terms of access to adequate amounts of PPE (protective equipment) and to testing. The aim was to make hospitals ready to receive an influx of expected COVID-19 patients. According to an Amnesty International Report 2020, the government had committed many abuses of human rights. The Scientific Advisory Group for Emergencies/SAGE published on 26 May 2022, its consensus statement which estimates that during the first 23 weeks of the pandemic – 4 March 2020 to 7 August 2020 – "there were

[11] There are no comparable figures for the UK as it does not collect such statistics in terms of age – see Webb, 2021 for the technical difficulties in working out a reliable figure based on available data, although the evidence points to the following estimate: in age groups up to and including 60-69, fewer than 1 in 1,000 people have died from coronavirus; age 70-79, it is 2 in every 1,000; age 80-89, it is 7 in every 1,000 people and age 90 and over, it is 18 people in every 1,000 people. These estimates aligned with figures produced elsewhere world-wide.

about 29,542 excess deaths in all care homes in England" (see SAGE Report, 2022).

Conclusion

1 The exploration of this chapter confirms yet again that the Monogenic Conception of Disease (held as dogma) cannot account for disease-generation by simplistically picking out the coronavirus itself, SARS-CoV-2, as "the cause" of COVID-19.
2 Disease-generation is only adequately accounted for in terms of the **W**hat, **W**here, **W**hen and **W**ho questions and the interplay between them.
3 The relevance of these questions and the interconnectedness of their complexities is borne out by the fate of the group of the elderly (from 60 to over 80 in age) with its risk of infection as well as death in the pandemic. Their vulnerability can also only be fully explained by appealing to both Clinical Medicine and Epidemiology. In particular, the elderly in care homes are people who are frail physically in general, with specific co-morbidities (such as heart conditions, high blood pressure and so forth) and in some cases are also mentally fragile (a few even with Alzheimer's Dementia). The then UK government had been rightly condemned by Amnesty International, 2020 as having committed many abuses of human rights through a moral failure underpinned by a cognitive failure of understanding the nature of disease-generation and illness in society, especially during an epidemic/pandemic. The prediction of excess death (4 March 2020 to 7 August 2020) could have been made by anyone with common-sense on the grounds that the deliberate exposure of the fragile and the vulnerable with extant morbidities and other disadvantageous health conditions to a pathogenic virus could/would act as the proverbial straw that breaks the camel's back.

CHAPTER 5

"THE CAUSE" IN TERMS OF CONTROLLABILITY AND PREVENTABILITY

This chapter returns to the theme discussed in the preceding chapters, namely, the need to abandon the Monogenic Conception of Disease in terms of how it answers the **W**ho, **W**hat, **W**here and **W**hen questions (when it is understood simplistically and held as dogma). It bears repeating that the fault lies in its singling out from a set of causally relevant conditions the virus SARS-CoV-2, privileging it as "the cause" of COVID-19. It does so, as we have seen, by following the Henle-Koch postulates which uphold the key formula "one cause, one effect", where the cause, depending on the context, could be a bacterium, a virus, a gene, a fungus, a parasite, a prion.

This chapter looks at another criterion for assigning "the cause" or "the causes" of disease-generation, that expounded by Collingwood, which in brief may be formulated thus: single out as "the cause" or "causes" from a set of appropriate conditions which can successfully be used to control and/or prevent the disease at hand. Under a fortunate set of circumstances, medical experts (in Clinical Medicine as well as Epidemiology) could figure out which is the most effective measure to adopt to achieve the goal of controlling and/or preventing the disease or ameliorating its severity. These measures could be pharmaceutical in character (falling into the domain of Clinical Medicine) or non-pharmaceutical strategies (falling into the domain of Epidemiology). The term "effective" is used in this context to mean how many lives these measures might save in terms of deaths from COVID-19 per million or per 100,000 based on excess mortality in a pandemic period over earlier non-pandemic times.

Collingwood's Controllability Criterion

In Chapter 2, we have briefly introduced the concept of "inus conditions" advocated in Mackie, 1974. By this, Mackie meant that no single factor should be singled out as "the cause" as each of the several relevant factors identified, taken on its own, is neither necessary nor sufficient, although each is a necessary component of this particular sufficient complex of "inus conditions". Applied in the context of COVID-19, as the preceding chapters of this book have shown, any one case of infection cannot be explained in terms of the pathogenic agent, SARS-CoV-2. It is not a sufficient condition as it may be present but there may be no COVID-19 as happens in asymptomatic cases; we find it co-present with at least one or more other relevant conditions said to be conducive to disease-generation, such as age, health-status (whether there are co-morbidities or not), place and kind of employment, lifestyle characteristics such as diet, living conditions and so forth – these together constitute the "inus conditions".

On the other hand, is SARS-CoV-2, unproblematically, a necessary condition for the occurrence of COVID-19? In other words, if no SARS-CoV-2 is discovered in the person, then there is no infection, and hence the person is free of COVID-19. Unfortunately, things can get more complicated than this. We need to know how COVID-19 is identified? Is it identified via its characteristics in terms of its symptoms which are said to range from mild to severe and may include the following: fever or chills, coughs, shortness of breath or difficulty with breathing, fatigue, muscle or body aches, headache, new loss of taste or smell, sore throat, congestion or runny nose, nausea or vomiting, diarrhoea? Compare this list with a list for flu/influenza symptoms which include the following: fever, malaise, headache, runny nose, sneezing, reduced sense of smell, metallic taste in mouth, chills, cough, body pain or muscle pain, sore throat. What are the symptoms of cold? These are generally: runny or blocked nose, pain in the nose or sinus, sore throat, headache, cough, sneezing, fever and/or chills, muscle and body aches, tiredness.

Imagine yourself as a doctor and three patients present themselves: the first with the list of symptoms for COVID-19, the second for flu and the third for cold. How could the doctor be sure that it is COVID-19 and not flu, just based on studying the lists of symptoms? The obvious answer is that they cannot. What is resorted to are further diagnostic tests. These may yield results very quickly, in under 30 minutes in the case of flu although they may be unreliable as they may yield false positive or false negative results. Rapid lateral flow tests (RAT) for COVID-19 using swabs from throat or nose can deliver results between 10 and 30 minutes, depending on the type of tests. Such tests involve a high risk of giving a false negative result, telling you that you are free from the disease when you are not, as they involve more of the virus in your sample than is found in it in order to report a positive result. The gold standard for COVID-19 testing, as already mentioned in the last chapter, is the PCR lab-based test.

In other words, the medical profession does not rely on doctors looking at the list of symptoms to determine if the patient is suffering from COVID-19. It relies on identifying the virus, that is, the SARS-CoV-2 pathogen to do the job. This means that the disease is identified and defined in terms of the pathogenic cause. According to the Monogenic Conception of Disease, "the cause" of COVID-19 (the effect) is "SARS-CoV-2; according to data, "the cause" is part of "the effect"; cause and effect are not, therefore, two distinct and separate items or phenomena. This is a pretty bizarre conclusion for the Monogenic Conception of Disease, if the arguments presented against it are coherent. However, this criticism may not be fatal as empirically the two items or phenomena are distinct – COVID-19 the disease (the effect of the cause) is a set of symptoms, all observable and ascertainable while SARS-CoV-2 (the virus which is the cause of the effect) is also observable and ascertainable, albeit not by the naked eye but under the electron microscope and other lab tests. We are all by now very familiar with the image of the coronavirus, shown with its spikes poking out rather like the spikes of a hedgehog. Maybe it is time to leave aside the Monogenic Conception of Disease with its limitations (when held as a dogma) and in spite of its rich and impressive history.

The Monogenic Conception of Disease followed from the triumphalism of the Age of Bacteriology pioneered in the second half of the nineteenth century and brought to therapeutic fruition by the Age of Antibiotics in the second half of the twentieth century. This triumphalism, on the part of Clinical Medicine, enjoyed a second wave which arrived in the second half of the twentieth century when molecular genetics/biology was established, although it did not last very long as the results of the Human Genome Project completed at the beginning of this century put a damper on the view that genes simplistically could be privileged as "the cause" of disease-generation. The paradigm of Reductionism has begun to show some signs of losing its firm grip on scientific theory and its explanatory framework.

However, well before this glimmer of change on the horizon, the under-appreciated English philosopher (who was also a historian and an archaeologist), R. G. Collingwood (1889-1943) had analysed the notion of cause in his address to the Aristotelian Society in London in 1938. He distinguished between three senses of "cause," of which the second (which he called Sense II) is precisely about controllability. He also specifically mentioned that it is this understanding of cause with which medicine is most preoccupied. For this reason, it is appropriate to cite here, unapologetically, some key long passages from it (Collingwood 1938, 89-90):

> In Sense II … the word cause expresses an idea relative to human action; but the action is an action intended to control not other human beings (such as

> in Sense I), but things in "nature," or "physical" things. In this sense, the "cause" of an event in nature is the handle, so to speak, by which we can manipulate it. If we want to produce or to prevent such a thing, and cannot produce or eliminate it immediately (as we can produce or prevent certain movements of our own bodies), we set about looking for its "cause." The question "what is the cause of an event y?" means in this case "how can we produce or prevent y at will?" This sense of the word may be defined as follows. *A cause is an event or state of things which it is in our power to produce or prevent, and by producing or preventing we can produce or prevent that whose cause it is said to be. …*
>
> Suppose someone claimed to have discovered the cause of cancer, but added that his discovery though genuine would not in practice be of any use because the cause he had discovered was not a thing that could be produced or prevented at will. Such a person would be universally ridiculed and despised. No one would admit that he had done what he claimed to do. It would be pointed out that he did not know what the word cause (in the context of medicine, be it understood) meant. For in such a context a proposition of the form x causes y "implies the proposition" x is something that can be produced or prevented at will" as part of the definition of "cause." For in such a context a proposition of the form "x causes y" implies the proposition "x is something that can be produced or prevented at will" as part of the definition of "cause."

The first part of the second passage requires some special comment, which is to point out that Collingwood was wrong to imply that medicine is nothing but effective treatments/cures; that it has no legitimate interest in obtaining theoretical knowledge and understanding about the conjunction of causal factors leading to diseases. The truth which Collingwood had failed to comprehend and hence ignored is that medicine has a foot in both the scientific/theoretical and the therapeutic domains. Indeed, as the history of medicine shows, new therapies are increasingly expected to come from basic theoretical breakthroughs in the biomedical sciences. As already observed, the Human Genome Project and its related basic science, molecular genetics/biology are expected to play this critical role in the future. However, in spite of this flaw in Collingwood's one-sided account of medicine, his analysis of cause in Sense II in terms of controllability/preventability remains pertinent and insightful.

In any case, he correctly pointed out that this sense of cause belongs to practice, not theory. It belongs to what Aristotle called "practical science", where knowledge is not valued for its own sake, out of intellectual curiosity, but utility. It also sits comfortably with the Baconian view of science in particular (that knowledge is power, that nature is conquered by obeying her) and in general with the ideological goal of the modern project of science (and of medicine), that is, to use science in order to manipulate/control nature to suit our purposes.[1] Therefore, built into this sense of cause, is the idea that cause and effect are related in the way means and ends are related. When we single out a factor as the cause, we are saying in the practical/therapeutic context that it is the means by which we achieve the end of eradicating/ameliorating something deemed undesirable (such as pain, discomfort, death which go generally with diseases). The relationship between means and ends is about rationality as efficiency, what Kant called the hypothetical imperative [2] and what Habermas called instrumental rationality.[3]

Collingwood was also correct in pointing out that Sense II must be distinguished from Sense III [4] – the latter belongs to theoretical discourse, what we earlier have called the explanatory context. In this context, we have found Mackie's combination of factors, which he calls "inus conditions", to be appropriate. Sense II is not interested *per se* in "inus conditions", or in looking for all the other necessary conditions which may be jointly sufficient for the effect to occur; it simply assumes that they exist. Rather, it is interested *per se* in identifying as cause a factor the manipulation of which would lead to the desired outcome. Let us just mention one illustration in the recent history of medicine – the medical community was finally convinced that the bacterium, *H. pylori* is "the cause" of peptic ulcers when certain antibiotics were convincingly shown to have made a difference to significantly lowering the re-occurrence of the disease through the eradication of the bacterium. [5] Cause in Collingwood's Sense II is tied up with human agency, with action, with intervention rather than with mere observation of phenomena.

---

[1] For a detailed exploration of this thesis, see Lee, 2012.

[2] For a brief account, see Johnson and Cureton 2022.

[3] For a recent critical assessment, see Wedgewood 2011.

[4] Collingwood 1938, 97-8 writes that in this sense, "a cause is necessary (a) in its existence, as existing whether or no human beings want it to exist (b) in its operation, as producing its effects no matter what else exists or does not exist… The cause leads to its effect by itself, or 'unconditionally'; in other words the relation between cause and effect is one-one relation… "

[5] For details, see Lee, 2012, 144-145; in some cases, the infection can be removed by using an antibiotic such as tinidazole.

How to Control/Prevent/Ameliorate the Incidence of COVID-19

As above brief account has made clear, Collingwood's criterion in terms of cause as controllability is agnostic as to what the measure is, whether it falls into Clinical Medicine or Epidemiology. The only pertinent question to raise is this: does it work? Is it truly effective in controlling or preventing the undesirable effect from occurring?

In the domain of Clinical Medicine, the following measures have been advocated and invoked (see Auwaerter and Casadevall 2022), none of which is established as a "magic bullet", though some of them have limited efficacy:

(a) Antiviral pills for patients at high risk of severe infection or with other indications for this treatment. Antiviral drugs do not kill the virus but decrease the production of new viruses inside host cells – in this way, they can shorten the duration of the illness and also reduce complications for the patients. Two such pills, available only as prescribed medicines, for those considered to be at high risk of progressing to severe COVID-19, to be swallowed are called Paxlovid and Molnupiravir – the US Food and Drug Administration/FDA had granted an emergency use authorisation/EUA in December 2021 for patients who satisfied certain specified criteria in terms of age (at least 12 years old), weight (at least 88 lbs), tested positive for COVID-19, had co-morbidities such as cancers, diabetes, obesity. Paxlovid should not be taken by patients who were taking some other medications such as certain blood thinners and immunosuppressants. In some cases, COVID-19 could come back after treatment with Paxlovid – such patients should re-isolate for at least five days until fever had subsided and symptoms had improved.

(b) Patients deemed serious enough to be admitted to hospitals were prescribed the antiviral drug Remdesivir, originally developed to treat people infected with the Ebola and hepatitis C viruses. This drug was intravenously prescribed.

(c) Monoclonal antibodies, which are manufactured in laboratories, had been prescribed for some patients through infusion into the bloodstream. However, in January 2022, the US CDC discontinued this form of therapy as it was not found, in general, to have been effective with recent coronavirus variants, although, the US National Institutes of Health still sanctioned the use of a particular monoclonal antibody called bebtelovimab, for patients aged 12 and over, but only when Paxlovid and Remdesivir were not clinically appropriate for such patients.

(d) In June 2021, the US FDA granted an EUA for Tocilizumab for adults and children hospitalised with severe COVID-19. This is a biologic agent approved originally to treat autoimmune illnesses such as rheumatoid arthritis. It was given by medical practitioners either as an injection or infusion. [6]

In the domain of non-pharmaceutical/Epidemiological measures, these range from: keeping physical/social distance, avoiding crowded spaces, meeting others outdoors rather than indoors, mask-wearing in public, ensuring adequate ventilation in indoor spaces, testing-tracking-tracing in domestic context as well as in that of international travel at points of entry, self-isolating if tested positive but also when symptoms were mild, lockdown of cities/regions/countries, pursuing a zero-COVID-19 policy.[7] These strategies all had economic costs and are heavily value-laden in character – this aspect will be explored later in particular (Chapter 8) in the context of geopolitics.

Conclusion

1 This chapter wishes to present the Collingwood Criterion of Controllability/Preventability as an alternative guide to action from the methodological vantage point – it permits one to single out one or more of Mackie's "inus conditions" to cope with the viral phenomenon.
2 Collingwood's Controllability/Preventability Criterion cuts across the Clinical Medicine–Epidemiology divide, as it is applicable to either domain. Which measure is better at prevention/control is then simply a matter of assessing the relevant empirical data available.
3 Indeed, there is at least one measure which can be clearly identified and shown to fall into both domains of biomedicine, Clinical Medicine and Epidemiology. This is vaccines and vaccination, which Chapter 6 will explore.

[6] See "Covid Therapeutics" n.d. which counsels caution on the part of doctors in the use of such drugs.
[7] Or one of co-existing with the virus – see Normile 2022. See also Kucharski 2022.

CHAPTER 6

COVID-19, VACCINES AND VACCINATION: WHAT THEY TEACH US ABOUT THE NATURE OF MEDICINE, ILLNESS AND SOCIETY

This chapter may be read as a sequel to Lee 2019 published in *Synthese* about Epidemiology but which was written well before the emergence of the epidemic/pandemic called COVID-19 today. "Patient zero" of COVID-19 was said to be someone identified in Wuhan, China on 8 December 2019, although in reality, such a patient may never be identified. [1] However, on 30 December 2019, a hospital in Wuhan had confirmed a new type of coronavirus which was reported to the World Health Organisation/WHO. On 11-12 January 2020, Chinese scientists had sequenced the virus's genome. The virus, named SARS-CoV-2, has turned out to involve a succession of variants since then. Alpha (B.1.1.7) with samples first documented in the UK, September 2020; Beta (B.1.351) in South Africa, May 2020; Delta (B.1.617.2) in India, October 2020 and Omicron (B.1.1.529) in multiple countries, 26 November 2021. These labels/names are constructed by the WHO's Technical Advisory Group on SARS-CoV-2 Virus Evolution/TAG-VE. Some data is now available about the impact of these variants. Furthermore, vaccines have been developed in record time and vaccination has and is being carried out world-wide. This is, therefore, a suitable moment to assess the validity of the theoretical framework proposed in my 2019 paper. The critical assessment in this book focuses on the concept of the vaccine to test that framework. The outcome is a positive one.

It is standardly understood in biomedicine that there are two domains: Epidemiology and Clinical Medicine. The former is concerned with non-pharmaceutical measures in the control of disease, the latter with pharmaceutical interventions. However, Epidemiology is commonly considered to play the role of Cinderella to Clinical Medicine as

[1] A study shows that SARS-CoV-2 was circulating in Northern Italy since December 2019 – see La Rosa, Mancini, Ferraro, *et al.* 2021.

methodologically it cannot satisfy the gold standard of mounting Randomised Controlled Trials/RCT. [2] Yet, looking critically at data which have emerged in the present COVID-19 pandemic, it is not obvious that the gap between these two domains cannot be challenged, especially in the context of assessing the role of vaccines in controlling the transmission of infection. Vaccines typically constitute a pharmaceutical intervention and, therefore, fall under Clinical Medicine. Yet the outcome of vaccination is not simply studied and measured in clinical terms, such as the level of antibodies against the prevailing variant of SARS-CoV-2 in the individual pre and post infection, how much brain shrinkage infection can cause to the brain, ascertainable via brain scans pre and post infection, or how anxious or worried a person is about being jabbed by a vaccination. It is also studied epidemiologically. For instance, are front-line workers (nurses, doctors, ambulance personnel and others), low-paid workers, people belonging to certain groups (Black, Asian and Minority Ethnic in the UK), people with co-morbidities more likely to be infected than those who do not belong to them? Such investigations are typically epidemiological in character.

In other words, to do justice to the present pandemic, one must challenge this division of labour between Clinical Medicine and Epidemiology. This chapter presents a more comprehensive analytical framework for understanding the COVID-19 phenomenon. It argues that Epidemiological Thinking, far from being "inferior"/ "substandard" is the way forward – that all domains of Medical Thinking must be understood in terms of the complicated network of conceptual and causal relationships between the virus/bacteria, the person who succumbs to the virus (the patient), the treatment (vaccine) prescribed for the patient, the doctor, the research scientist in the labs, the Epidemiologist who studies disease patterns rather than individual patients, the community out there in which the person affected by the disease lives and forms a part, and so forth. Epidemiological Thinking is bidirectional, multifactorial and, hence, Wholist, not Reductionist. And so is Medical Thinking in the two domains of Clinical Medicine and Epidemiology.

Vaccines: Striding the Clinical Medicine-Epidemiological Divide

Vaccines have a foot in either camp. The concept of vaccine is unintelligible and practically inoperable unless it is seen to play a role in both Clinical Medicine and Epidemiology. In the history of vaccine production, vaccines to control COVID-19 have appeared in record time – the first to appear in

---

[2] For a detailed critique of these claims, see Lee, 2012, 158-174, and Lee 2017a.

the West on 11/12/2020 was the Pfizer-BioNTech vaccine, just under a year after the genome of SARS-CoV-2 was completed by Chinese scientists and made known to other scientists world-wide (on 07/01/2020). In China, their two first vaccines were revealed to the world in September 2020. [3] The fastest development prior to the COVID-19 vaccines was that for mumps in 1967 which took four years.

Everything happened at an unprecedented break-neck speed. As already observed, so-called "Patient zero" was identified in Wuhan, China on 08/12/2019; by 30/12/2019, the Jinyintan Hospital in Wuhan, using the RT-PCR test had confirmed a new type of coronavirus in a patient with strange pneumonia. By 11/01/2020, the WHO had received information from the Chinese scientists as well as the Chinese government that the virus's genome had been sequenced.

The successful sequencing of the virus's genome is critical to the manufacture of COVID-19 vaccines, especially the mRNA varieties. Such sequencing is a lab-based activity and so is the development of the vaccines based on the understanding it provides. Therefore, they belong firmly to the domain of Clinical Medicine. However, that is only one side of the story; the other side belongs to the domain of Epidemiology when the vaccines produced in laboratories have to be tested against the most extensive recruitment of trial-participants during Phase IV of the vaccine-testing. Epidemiology kicks in to help identify as many potential confounding variables as possible so that they would be eliminated and not undermine the results of the test – this means how to recruit the right groupings to take part in the trial. In other words, one could argue that RCTs, the gold standard of Clinical Medicine cannot do without an input from Epidemiology in the attempt to identify and avoid confounding variables.

Furthermore, Epidemiology attempts to understand in subtler details how different groupings in society may react to vaccines, not only during trials but when they are released as safe, secure and effective against the disease. Take this example. In the UK, it was said that some members of the

---

[3] The Western ones, namely, Pfizer-BioNTech and the Moderna vaccines use mRNA whereas the Chinese ones (Sinopharm and Sinovac) use the traditional inactivated virus. Accessed January 13, 2022. https://www.nature.com/ articles/ d41586-021-01146-0 ; https://www.medicalnewstoday. com/ articles/how-did-we-develop-a-covid-19-vaccine-so-quickly (undated but cannot be earlier than November 2021; "A Timeline of COVID-19 Vaccine Development" | BioSpace (3 December 2020); https://www.nature.com/ articles/d41586-021-01146-0 ; "China's COVID vaccines are going global — but questions remain" (see *Nature* 2021 (May 4); "China shows off COVID-19 vaccines for first time" (see *Medical Xpress* 2020 (7 September)).

Muslim community were resistant to vaccination although Islam, as a religion, is not in principle against vaccines and vaccination. So where did the resistance come from? It turned out that some members of the Muslim community had numerous worries and anxieties of which a crucial one was whether the manufacture of the vaccines involves a material or process which was *haram*, that is, not *halal*. Was porcine DNA involved at some stage of the manufacturing process? The imams in the mosques had to address such suspicions and others based on myths and "fake news" (such as people could be "tagged" during vaccination, that the vaccines could modify a person's DNA in the case of those vaccines which use the mRNA technology).[4] The clerics not only reassured their flock that the vaccines are above such suspicion and anxiety but also that as Muslims they have a duty to prevent harm to others. Members of the UK Muslim community who are prone to take on board such suspicions and rumours are, on the whole, not as well educated as their fellow Muslims who do not subscribe to such "fake news". It was fitting that the imams addressed these issues during their Friday sermons.[5]

To put things in a nutshell, to tackle COVID-19, one needs a comprehensive, all-encompassing orientation which looks at the viral disease/illness not simply from the vantage point of laboratory science or even of Clinical Medicine but also from that of Epidemiology, of disease/illness understood as a phenomenon occurring in society affecting specific people both as members of groups and as individuals in specific ways.[6]

---

[4] Accessed June 21, 2022. https://www.theguardian.com/world/2021/jan/14/ imams-mosques-uk-reassure-muslim-worshippers-covid-vaccines.

[5] Another example of how ethnicity could affect the practice of Clinical Medicine in the UK. The charity Alzheimer's Society has published a report (Gregory 2022) that people from South Asian communities (the term "South Asian" in this context, in the main, refers to people who come from or whose parents come from India, Pakistan and Bangladesh) fear stigma and taboo which follow from a diagnosis of dementia. Such families, therefore, do not step forward readily to seek diagnosis and help. People with such a background also, unfortunately, are at higher risk of other illnesses such as heart disease, stroke and diabetes. Such co-morbidities increase the likelihood of dementia.

[6] The UK is currently (as reported in February 2023) conducting a public inquiry into COVID-19 – see Livingston and Cainer 2022. Nearly all minority ethnic groups are urging the inquiry to look into the role played by structural racism in the pandemic. They want an explanation of "why the death toll was significantly higher among the Black and minority ethnic community." For instance, the mortality rate for Bangladeshi males was three times that for white British males while that for

The Pyramid of Evidence Framing the Clinical Medicine-Epidemiological Divide

Table 6.1 below presents this framing, though not in the standard format of a triangle or pyramid.

Level l The Gold Standard	Evidence from one or more Randomised Controlled Trials (RCTs)
Level ll	ll.1 Evidence from Controlled Trials without Randomisation
	ll.2 Evidence from Cohort or Case-Control Analytic Studies
	ll.3 Evidence from multiple Time Series Observational Studies
Level lll	Opinions of respected authorities built upon vast clinical experience, descriptive studies, reports of expert committees
Level lV	Anecdotal evidence based on one person's experience only

Table 6.1 Table of Medical Evidence (more familiarly presented as The Pyramid of Evidence) invoked today – if higher or the highest level (Level I) is not available, then move down to the next best level

As set out clearly above, the highest level of probity is occupied by evidence based on RCTs.[7] This discussion is meant to be brief, not comprehensive, and serves simply to highlight for the reader the fact that evidence from Epidemiology is assigned to Level ll and its three sub-divisions, and that the "real mark of Cain" worn by Epidemiology is that it fails to satisfy not so much the criterion of being a controlled test but that of randomisation. The technique of randomisation makes eminent sense in Clinical Medicine, as it is concerned crucially with pharmaceutical measures of controlling a

Pakistani women was twice that for white British women, according to the Office for National Statistics.

[7] This is not the place to critically assess this prestigious claim made on behalf of RCTs – for details of such exploration, see sources already cited.

disease, namely, drugs (primarily in the form of pills) considered to be truly effective in terms alone of their pharmaceutical potency (the active ingredients of a drug) rather than a reliance on the so-called placebo effect. Randomisation, including the use of double-blinding, is then considered as critical to the control and elimination of the placebo effect.

In 1906, Theodore Roosevelt, President of the USA passed the first Food and Drug Act/FDA. This provided an important framework eventually a half century later for the pharmaceutical manufacturers to become what today some people call "Big Pharma" with its deep pockets and immense lobbying power after the end of WWII, cementing the emergence of the golden age of antibiotics. In Phase III of a drug trial as conducted by a pharmaceutical company, the new drug is given to some patients with the disease for which the treatment is targeting using the RCT-Model of Testing – should the drug perform better (in an acceptable statistical sense of that term), then the FDA would license the company to sell it. Phase III preceded by Phase I and II are said between them to warrant a sufficient degree of safety and effectiveness. However, it is only in Phase IV when the drug is released on the public that real testing begins as it alone satisfies the methodological requirement of large numbers of participants in order to be meaningful.

In spite of the gold standard status of the RCT, it is well to bear the following points in mind:

(a) Not every treatment requires the *imprimatur* of the RCT – in cases where the effects, say, of a drug are so obvious in immediately lowering mortality, no RCT is required. This was the case with sulphonamide and penicillin. [8]
(b) Not every new treatment could/would be subjected to RCTs on practical grounds, as there are far too many such treatments, continuously introduced into the market, by pharmaceutical companies, which differ from extant products, seemingly, in small ways. [9]

---

[8] Cochrane, 1972, 22.

[9] The operative word "seemingly" is this author's own gloss. It is to draw attention to the fact that as no RCT would or could be expected for such products, there is no evidence either way as to whether such small variations in their chemical composition would produce different effects from their prototypes for which the RCT had been conducted. This default axiom, undoubtedly, is economically and practically sound, but is it also methodologically sound? There may be room for some doubt regarding the latter aspect – see following footnote for more details.

(c) One should distinguish between two different contexts in which RCTs are mounted – by the pharmaceutical industry and by the medical community which uses pharmaceutical products in treating patients.

This discussion here only comments on point (c) above, to show that the main aim of conducting RCTs in the two contexts is different. Pharmaceutical companies are primarily interested in getting past the licensing legislation as laid out, for instance, in the US Pure Food and Drug Act or their equivalents in other, by and large, developed economies. Consequently, their remit is somewhat limited – all that a RCT needs to demonstrate is that the product can perform in the way the label claims it does. For instance, a drug ultimately to be marketed (and patented) to treat depression must be backed by some evidence that it does have some effect in alleviating depression. It is not part of the remit of such trials to ensure how effective in reality it is compared to other drugs, or how safe it is in the longer run. It is unfortunate that the public and, indeed, even some health professionals, mistakenly, believe that the licensing authorities are concerned, in particular, with health and safety of the public. [10]

As already mentioned, the true effects of a new drug cannot be ascertained by RCTs conducted by pharmaceutical companies, as these trials necessarily have a short time limit; assessing the true impact from the health and safety points of view comes from long-term monitoring of the effects of a new drug when released for general use. This was indeed how the very serious side effects of the drug, thalidomide, were ultimately discovered. In the light of that catastrophe, guidelines for drug testing/use have been tightened, but when all is said and done, the ultimate "guinea pigs" are the patients in the world at large who take the drug which their doctors prescribe for them. Strategies for long term monitoring have been devised, such as the yellow card scheme – for instance, the scheme in the UK is operated by the Medicines and Healthcare Products Regulatory Agency/ MHRA which encourages not only health professionals but also members of the public to report to the Agency any side effects (adverse drug reactions) of a drug or vaccine so that it can identify previously unidentified safety issues.[11]

---

[10] See Healy 2009; Silverman, 1985, 151. Dr Patrick Vallance, Head of Drug Discovery of GSK (GlaxoSmithKline) in 2010 was reported as saying that (a) clinical trials involve at best thousands of cases, but the true side effects require hundreds of thousands of cases; (b) therefore no drug is totally safe and uncertainty is built into the matter – see BBC Two Horizon (Pill Poppers), 2010; Angell 2004.

[11] Accessed June 12, 2022. http://yellowcard.mhra.gov.uk/ .

There are two main justifications for the use of RCTs in the wider context of medical practice in society at large, which appear to be closely related: (a) whether the latest new treatment promoted by the pharmaceutical industry is more or less efficacious than the extant standard treatment(s); (b) as the latest product is often more expensive than the older options (especially in cases where patent rights have lapsed), is it cost-effective to endorse prescription of the former when money is always (relatively) in short supply? It is in this spirit that the National Institute for Health and Clinical Excellence /Nice [12] was set up in the UK in April 1999 whose main remit is to draw up guidelines about the use of a range of drugs.

Conclusion

This chapter demonstrates that the data appear to show that the SARS-CoV-2/COVID-19 phenomenon falls under the domain not only of Clinical Medicine but also that of Epidemiology. It demonstrates this by focussing on vaccines/vaccination which superficially is understood merely as a clinical, pharmaceutical measure but in reality, is also an Epidemiological (that is to say, a non-pharmaceutical) intervention. In other words, an all-round Wholist orientation is called for in understanding the nature of the present epidemic/pandemic.

If the arguments presented for this approach are coherent and survive critical scrutiny, then, ironically, its methodology is shown to approximate more to that of Epidemiology than to what underpins Clinical Medicine (as standardly theorised under the Monogenic Conception of Disease). Earlier chapters have established that this conception (which is held as dogma) adheres to a simplistic unidirectional, monofactorial model of causality whereas the causal model underlying Epidemiological Thinking is bi-directional and multifactorial. The differences between the two models will be further explored in the following chapter, Chapter 7.

In other words, the points above may be made by saying that both domains can be adequately and fruitfully analysed within the framework of Ecosystem Thinking or Ecosystem-nesting. The next chapter explores this Wholist theme in some detail.

---

[12] It may be seen as a belated attempt to seriously implement the goal of efficiency advocated by Cochrane, 1972.

CHAPTER 7

ECOSYSTEM THINKING IS EPIDEMIOLOGICAL THINKING WHICH IS MEDICAL THINKING

This chapter explores the interconnectedness of the following themes in medicine today:

1 In spite of the fact that biomedicine has two main domains, namely, Clinical Medicine and Epidemiology, it turns out upon scrutiny that the thinking is similar, contrary to the standard orthodox understanding of these two domains.
2 The mode of understanding the nature of disease/illness whether in an individual patient or in groups of people in society at large in an epidemic/pandemic is more similar to Epidemiological Thinking than it is to Clinical Thinking which upholds the Monogenic Conception of Disease (held as dogma), critiqued in earlier chapters (2, 3 and 4).
3 Epidemiological Thinking may more insightfully be called Ecosystem Thinking which can be represented in terms of Ecosystem-nesting as concentric circles.
4 Ecosystem Thinking is offered as a research analytical tool, which could be used in contexts other than this one of understanding the SARS-CoV-2/COVID-19 epidemic/pandemic.

The Epidemiological Mode of Causal and Ecosystem Thinking

Clinical Medicine which relies on Randomised Controlled Trials as the main tool to ensure its privileged status at Level 1 in the Pyramid of Evidence (see Table 6.1) in turn relies on a particular model of causality to back it up. This model is what may be called the unidirectional, monofactorial model of causality/UMC, where there is one cause leading to one effect, thus:

Cause (Before) ——————————▶ Effect (After)

Figure 7.1 Simple Unidirectional, Monofactorial Causality

Figure 7.2 below represents a more complicated variant. A (the cause) leads to B (the effect), B in turn acts as the cause leading to the effect C, and so on along the chain.

Cause ——▶ Cause/ Effect ——▶ Cause/ Effect ——▶ Effect

Figure 7.2 A Series of Linked Cause and Effect

However, the two variants confirm that this kind of causation embodies two significant features:

(a) The causal arrow is unidirectional, from Cause to Effect.
(b) Causation is monofactorial, that is, only one causal variable is involved leading to one effect.

However, it is important to note that UMC does not underpin what has been called the Classical Version of the Monogenic Conception of Disease when Koch (following Pasteur) said that the cause of tuberculosis is the tubercle bacterium. Today, however, when the Monogenic Conception of Disease is held as dogma, it runs the risk in the case of COVID-19 of implying the UMC when it pronounces that the cause of COVID-19 is the virus, SARS-CoV-2 with its variants (when in reality it is only entitled to refer to "the cause" in terms of necessary condition, not of both necessary and sufficient conditions).[1]

In contrast, as shown in the case of vaccines, Epidemiology is more aware of the complexities of the causal scene. It does not subscribe either to the Monogenic Conception of Disease (held as dogma) or to the UMC but to the multifactorial model, in which more than one variable is at work in producing a disease pattern in society. That is why in Epidemiological Thinking, the causal arrow is bidirectional, not unidirectional, and is multifactorial, which involves what may be called the bidirectional, multifactorial mode of causality/BMC, thus:

---

[1] Refer back to earlier Chapters 2, 3 and 4 for a detailed account of these development and for a critique of the MCD (held as dogma).

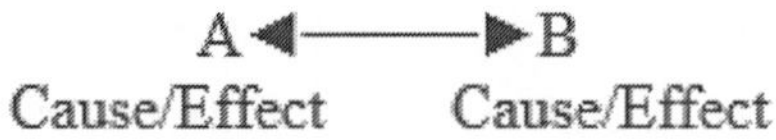

Figure 7.3 Causal arrow can be bidirectional.

In other words, phenomenon A causes B, the Effect, which in turn can causally affect A. To illustrate how this concept can be seen at work in Nature at large, imagine a hairline crack occurring in a rock – this is phenomenon A. Water enters the crack – this is phenomenon B. One can plausibly say that the existence of the crack (A) causes water (B/Effect) to enter the crack. B in turn causes the crack to widen a little. In other words, A and B are mutually Cause and Effect. Here is an illustration in the context of disease and disease-pattern occurring in society: the diagnosis of lung cancer would cause anxiety in the patient. In his anxiety the patient reaches out for his cigarettes. The consumption of such cigarettes has in the first place caused his lung cancer. Here is a mutually reinforcing relation between Cause and Effect.

The causal model invoked by this kind of epidemiological research (in the context of tobacco smoking and lung cancer) implies a more sophisticated variant of Epidemiological Thinking which may be represented by the image of the Triangle of Causation,[2] but greatly enhanced, as shown below:

[2] See Bhopal, 2008, 131-35. For the dimension of mathematical modelling in Epidemiology as pioneered by the nineteenth century epidemiologist, Ronald Ross (1857-1932) and the mathematician, Hilda Hudson, see Kucharski 2020. Ross was awarded the Nobel Prize in medicine in 1902 for his discovery in 1897 that malaria in humans was transmitted through the bite of infected anopheline mosquitoes, in particular of *P. falciparum.*

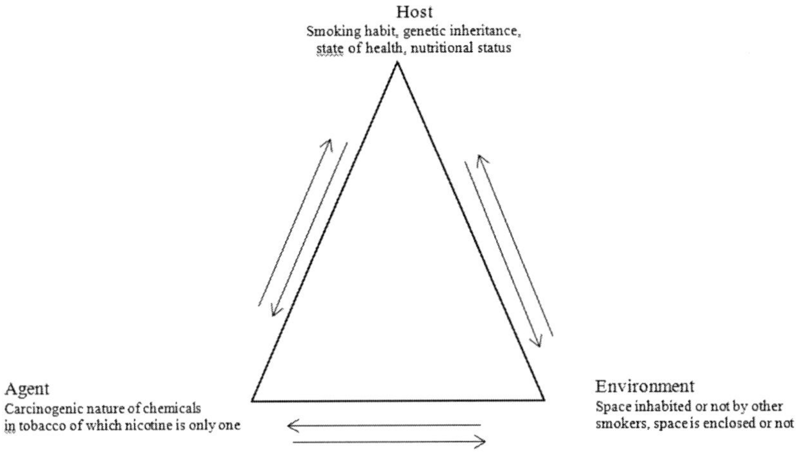

Figure 7.4 Epidemiological (enhanced) triangle of relevant variables and causation

There are three main variables: Host, Agent and Environment between which the causal arrows indicate reciprocity. This advanced causal model obviously differs from that exhibited by the Monogenic Conception of Disease (when held as dogma) and its UMC.

Note that in the smoking-lung cancer example not only is it the case that there are three main variables involved in the model of causation, but that each of these three main variables is internally complex.[3]

Host includes several variables, such as the smoking and/or the alcohol drinking habits of the individuals, their respective genetic inheritances, general state of their health/age/nutritional status/occupational status.

Agent includes the carcinogenic nature of not only one chemical, but also the many chemicals found in tobacco smoke, of which nicotine is only one.

Environment includes whether the space in which the individuals dwell/work consists of smokers, even if they themselves do not smoke, whether the space is enclosed or not, and if enclosed whether adequate

[3] This is what is meant by "multifactorial" in this context. It does not mean plural causes which obtain in cases when an effect is brought about by more than one cause acting independently of each other. For instance, peptic ulcer can be caused by either *Helicobacter pylori* or the overuse of NSAIDS – see Chapter 2.

ventilation obtains, and if not enclosed, whether the air outside is polluted or clean, and so on.

Of late, some researchers appear to want to develop this more nuanced characterisation of Epidemiology Thinking even further, to approximate it closer to Systems Thinking (of which Epidemiological Thinking is an exemplar). O'Connor and McDermott, 1997 distinguish a system from a heap: the former is a series of interconnected parts, which function as a Whole – when parts are removed or added to, it changes. Its behaviour depends on its overall structure (the arrangements of its component parts). The latter is a mere collection of its parts. Its parts function independently of one another, hence the arrangement of its components as well as overall structure are irrelevant. Its behaviour depends merely on its size.

The notion of system can be used to describe complex biological relationships (such as in Ecology, the study of ecosystems). It may be used to characterise relationships/processes found in an organisation, such as a company. It may also be used in understanding illnesses, their diagnoses and treatments as found in Classical Chinese Medicine.[4] Hence, this author prefers to call Systems Thinking Ecosystem Thinking (the reasons for doing so will become clearer in a moment).

Ecosystem Thinking as Systems Thinking is keen to point out that the relationship between events/processes involves complicated systemic linkages, drawing out clearly such a methodological implication of Wholism. One can re-cast the enhanced Triangle of Causation in terms of nesting ecosystems as shown in Figure 7.5 below: the Host (the person) as Ecosystem 1, the Agent (the chemicals in tobacco smoke which are carcinogenic to the Host) as Ecosystem 2, the Environment as Ecosystem 3. Indeed, 1, 2 and 3 may be said to form another more-encompassing ecosystem, namely, Ecosystem 4.

---

[4] See Hejazi, n.d.; Lee, 2017, 21, 126-132, 138, 311, 325.

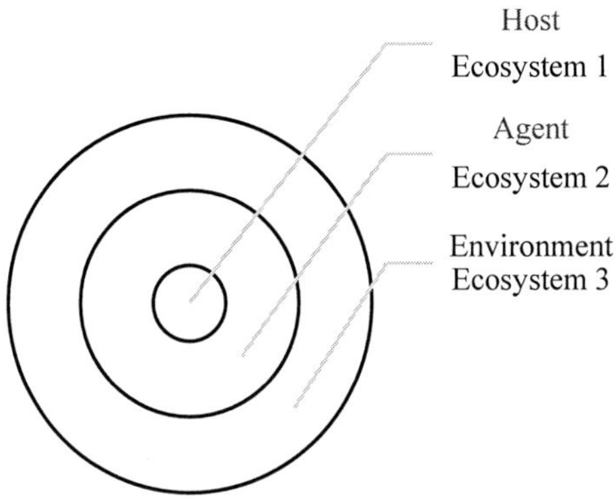

Figure 7.5 Epidemiological causation to Ecosystem-nesting of concentric circles

The most important aspect of Systems Thinking which have impressed researchers working at the cutting edge of Epidemiological Thinking is that "from a systems perspective, health is conceptualized as an emergent property of a system, in which processes operating at the levels of individuals and populations are inextricably connected" (Diez Roux 2011, 1627-1634). Systems approaches emphasise the need to understand dynamic interrelations between various components.

> Because the effect of a given input depends on other conditions in the system, emphasis shifts from isolating the causal effect of a single factor to comprehending the functioning of the system as a whole. Complex systems typically include heterogeneous agents at various levels, contact structures between agents, adaptation, nonlinear dynamics, and stochasticity. These features lead to the emergence of patterns at various scales. (Diez Roux 2011)

Such an approach involves identifying and studying the presence of important causal loops in the system. In many types of population health problems, feedback mechanisms are found between behavioural and environmental features as well as between health and social circumstances. An instance of the former is this: the availability of healthy food promotes a healthier diet, which in turn creates an increase in the demand for healthy foods; an instance of the latter obtains when health affects income and income in turn affects health. These are self-reinforcing tendencies.

Enlarging a little: Take the case of the incidence of smoking, and ultimately of its related problems of disease and ill health and attempts to lower it. Admittedly, each of the following interventions produces some effect, each in its own right: smoking cessation programmes, prohibiting smoking in public spaces, increasing cigarette taxes, social marketing, and so on. However, the Epidemiologist in accordance with Systems Thinking would also consider what would happen when all the relevant interventions are combined; the total joint effect might be greater than the sum of their effects when produced in isolation from one another (synergistic effects). Changes within a system in a factor/variable providing feedback into the process may produce positive or negative impacts. Suppose high taxes on cigarettes would reduce the number of smokers. The next step to pursue is to see if higher taxation would lead to changes over time in social attitudes to smoking, which may then make it possible to increase enforcement of public smoking regulations. If it does, then this would be a positive feedback impact. On the other hand, raising cigarette taxes would mean the treasury has less money to render smoking cessation programmes accessible to help individuals to quit the habit. This then would lead to a negative feedback impact.

In other words, Systems Thinking embodies Wholism whose processes constitute a dynamic system with very intricate feedback loops, which can reinforce the processes of change or dampen them. Under the former, a new equilibrium would eventually be reached; under the latter, equilibrium would be restored. Wholism accommodates both instability and stability; both positive and negative feedback loops can occur in a system.

Epidemiological Thinking, Systems Thinking and Ecosystem Thinking (which this author prefers to argue for and use) belong to the family of models in causal thinking which emphasises an interconnectivity between the different parts of the system adding up to a coherent Whole. Ecosystem Thinking in terms of Ecosystem-nesting will provide the appropriate analytical framework for Epidemiology as well as Clinical Medicine by focussing on the embeddedness of vaccines and vaccination (as discussed in Chapter 6) in this nesting, which Figure 7.6 below is intended to demonstrate.

Before proceeding further, one must add the caveat that only ten concentric circles are drawn in this figure entirely for convenience. The actual number is up to those using the schema for their own purpose in hand. It could be less than ten or more than ten. The number is immaterial. An increase or decrease is justified entirely in terms of the context and the purpose served, as Ecosystem-nesting in terms of concentric circles is just a research analytical tool.

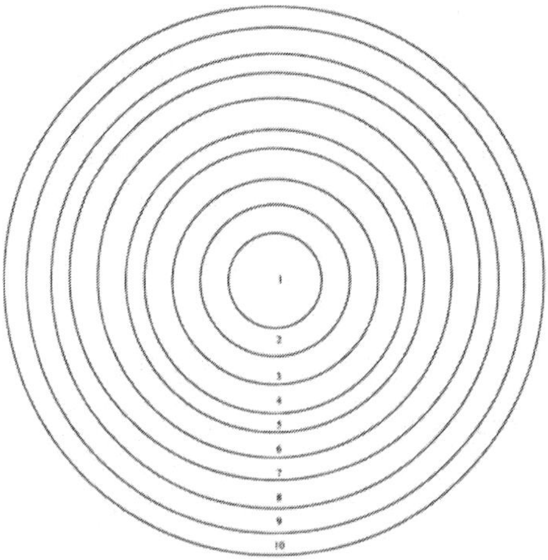

Figure 7.6 Ecosystem Thinking in terms of Ecosystem-*nesting* via concentric circles.

1 The genome of SARS-CoV-2 was quickly deciphered by the community of medical scientists by 11-12 January 2020, after a cluster of COVID-19 patients was identified in Wuhan, China in December 2019- January 2020.
2 SARS-CoV-2 is the virus identified under the Monogenic Conception of Disease (the Classical Version). However, it would not be correct to single it out without further qualification as the cause of COVID-19. To do so runs the risk of understanding the Monogenic Conception of Disease as dogma with its attendant UMC – the term "cause" under UMC refers to an understanding of it only as necessary condition, not as necessary and sufficient conditions. An adequate understanding of cause, however, requires identifying and grasping both conditions.
3 The virus (any virus), to replicate itself must enter an organism as it lacks the ability for replication otherwise. In this context, the animal is suspected to be a bat, a racoon dog or another animal not yet identified.
4 The virus in the infected animal in turn could enter the cells of another organism, thereby carrying on the transmission process.
5 This other organism infected in the transmission process could be a human who in turn infects other fellow humans.
6 Human beings are different from other organisms. Their unique kind of consciousness enables them to use language, to make abstractions and

inferences and to adhere to self-imposed norms in a self-conscious manner.

7 Human beings live in groups, clans, tribes, classes, underpinned generally by ethnicity, language, and/or religion, economic circumstances.
8 As such, the hopes, fears, anxieties, expectations (their psychology) are formed and informed by the social divisions listed at 7 above.
9 These tribes/ethnic groups/class/polity are embedded in the larger physical environment, in which they live and must survive (plants/animals/rivers/mountains or plains/climatic conditions/diseases).
10 Their social values (religious, cultural, economic, scientific) affect the way they regard the larger physical environment and their attitudes and their conduct to it.

Concentric circles or Ecosystems 1-5 fall, in the main, under the domain of Clinical Medicine, of lab science while concentric circles or Ecosystems 6-10 fall in general under the domain of Epidemiology, as Epidemiology studies disease patterns in different demographics in a society. Hence, one can also say that they fall under the domains of psychology, sociology, economics, politics, geopolitics, as all these spheres of activities affect disease patterns. Let us just cite some examples to make this point. Data show that economically developed, that is, rich countries suffer on the whole from disease conditions arising from obesity while developing or poor countries on the whole suffer from disease conditions arising from malnutrition or under-nutrition.[5] Within, say, a developed, rich country, its

---

[5] See https://worldpopulationreview.com/country-rankings/most-obese-countries; https://en.wikipedia.org/wiki/List_of_ countries by_GDP_(nominal) _per_capita. Accessed February 12, 2022. The second list gives figures for 216 countries listed in a descending order in terms of GDP per capita – on the whole, the richest countries (barring oil producing countries and those which operate as tax havens) are found in the West (position 1-18, interrupted at 4 by Bermuda; 21-30 (disrupted by Hong Kong at position 28); at the poor end, 144 -147, 166-170, 176-194 (interrupted by Pakistan at position 178), 197-216 (disrupted by North Korea at position 206 and Afghanistan at 207) are countries in Africa. In the list for obesity, the top ten positions are occupied by countries referred to as Oceania, with Nauru leading at 61.00% amongst adults and with Micronesia bringing up the rear at 45.80%. This specific list may be explained in terms of genetic factors in the population interacting with change from a traditional diet to a more Western one. (Europeans had first arrived during the sixteenth century. Colonisation by different European imperial powers occurred: the Spanish from the early seventeenth century, the Dutch, the British, the French, the German and the American in the nineteenth and twentieth centuries. Japan, too, muscled in at the beginning of WWl as well as during WWll.)

relatively poorer citizens live in areas more exposed to pollutants (such as particulates in the ambient atmosphere which are released by car traffic or neighbouring factories) and hence may suffer more from certain types of cancer correlated with such high exposure. [6] Their richer citizens tend to live in the so-called leafy suburbs where the air is cleaner, fresher and where trees and parks provide a salubrious physical and social environment to live and breathe. Furthermore, the residents tend to belong the AB, C1 categories (used by the UK Office for National Statistics).[7]

This system of social grading testifies amply to the fact that it has grasped that the psychology of an individual is formed and informed by their being a member of a group belonging to a certain social grade – their hopes and expectations as well as their fears and anxieties about their own future and that of their children are intimately tied up with a particular social grade. In other words, psychology cannot be grasped without grasping sociology, economics, politics, ethnicity and race. For instance, data on the whole show that those belonging to the AB social grade in the UK are mainly white and could be said to be Christian, no matter how attenuated their personal belief may be, while those belonging to grades DE tend to be non-white and/or immigrants or of immigrant-descent.[8]

Conclusion

The aim of this chapter is to demonstrate in brief how the COVID-19 data fit within the analytical framework of Epidemiology as Ecosystem Science originally proposed in the 2019 paper published by this author in *Synthese* before the emergence of COVID-19. Furthermore, very importantly, it goes one step further to argue that the data appear to show that the SARS-CoV-2/COVID-19 phenomenon falls under the domain not only of Epidemi-

---

Comparing the two lists shows a plausible link between obesity in Western countries and high GDP per capita in the same countries on the one hand, and on the other, another plausible link between the lower level of obesity in African countries and their low GDP per capita in the same countries. (See also "GDP Per Capita by Country in PPP Int$ Adjusted for Base Year and Informal Economy". Accessed September 22, 2022. https://www.worldometers. info/gdp/gdp-per-capita/).

[6] See, for example, Wong, Tsang, Lai, *et al.* 2016.

[7] AB as a social grade refers to higher and intermediate managerial, administrative, professional occupations while CI to supervisory, clerical and junior managerial, administrative, professional occupations. The remaining social grades are: C2 refers to skilled manual occupations; DE refer to semi-skilled and unskilled manual occupations, the unemployed belonging to these grades.

[8] This, however, is not to say that poor whites do not exist.

ology but also that of Clinical Medicine; that both domains can be adequately and fruitfully analysed within the framework of Ecosystem / Systems Thinking. It demonstrates this by focussing on vaccines and vaccination. Vaccination superficially is understood merely as a Clinical, pharmaceutical measure but in reality, is also an Epidemiological (that is to say, a non-pharmaceutical) intervention. (Refer back to Chapter 6.) In other words, an all-round Wholist orientation is called for in understanding the nature of the present epidemic/pandemic.

If the arguments presented for this approach are coherent and survive critical scrutiny, then, ironically, its methodology is shown to approximate more to that of Epidemiology than what underpins Clinical Medicine (as standardly theorised which rests on the Monogenic Conception of Disease, held as dogma) with its underlying UMC. In other words, Epidemiological Thinking is Medical Thinking which is Ecosystem Thinking. Ecosystem Thinking embodies Wholism and exemplifies the BMC (bidirectional, multifactorial) with their interconnected complexities between the various relevant factors as indicated by the data available concerning the generation of disease/illness in an individual and in society.

CHAPTER 8

COVID-19 AND MASK-WEARING: IN THE CONTEXT OF GEOPOLITICAL AND OTHER VALUES

One source offers this definition of "epidemic": "(it) refers to an increase, often sudden, in the number of cases of a disease above what is normally expected in that population in that area." The same source offers this definition of "pandemic": "Pandemic refers to an epidemic that is spread over several countries or continents, usually affecting a large number of people." [1] COVID-19, by 4-5 January 2020. satisfies this definition of an epidemic with its epicentre at Wuhan-Hubei, China when the World Health Organisation/WHO first announced the epidemic via Twitter and then official notification. The WHO's director-general, Dr Tedros Adhanom Ghebreyesus, however, on 30 January 2020 declared not a pandemic, but a PHEIC ("a public health emergency of international concern") when by that date, outside China, 83 cases in 18 countries had reported human-to-human transmission though with no deaths. It was not, however, till 11 March 2020 when Dr Tedros used the term "pandemic" instead of "PHEIC". It is plausible to explain his reluctance to call the viral phenomenon a pandemic for fear of causing unnecessary panic amongst the peoples and countries in the world. Whatever his motive, it would not be identical to that of the then US president, Donald Trump who initially denied outright the existence of the illness and/or downplayed its seriousness since report of the first case of COVID-19 in the USA on 21 January 2020. [2]

On 23 January 2020, the Chinese government imposed a lockdown on Wuhan and other cities; at the same time, it announced the building of new hospitals (called Fangcang hospitals) dedicated to the treatment of COVID-19 patients, the first of which was opened on 3 February 2020. By 26

---

[1] See "Epidemic, Endemic, Pandemic: What are the Differences?" 2021. However, on the terms themselves "PHEIC" and "pandemic", see earlier Chapter 4 for their clarification.

[2] See Timeline of Trump's Coronavirus Responses 2022.

January 2020, medical personnel and resources as well as food and volunteers from all over China had arrived in Wuhan to help the city. On 30 January 2020, China reported to the WHO 7,711 confirmed and 12,167 suspected cases – of the confirmed cases, 1,370 were severe with 170 deaths and 124 having recovered and discharged from hospital. Between 5 and 10 February 2020, more medical resources were sent to Hubei – 19 other provinces partnered with 16 Hubei cities rendering assistance. On 10 March 2020, the situation had so improved that all Fangcang hospitals were suspended as these became surplus to requirement.

On 26 February 2020, the WHO announced that daily new cases outside China exceeded those inside, with 2,790 cases across 37 counties and 44 deaths. On 8 April 2020, the lockdown of Wuhan officially ended. According to one estimate published by *The British Medical Journal* on 11/02/ 2021, Wuhan accounted for 3870 deaths out of a total of 4600 in China with 80,000 infected of which Wuhan had c 50,000. Lockdown apart, the measures adopted by Wuhan-China included: active case surveillance, rapid case diagnosis and management, strict follow-up, quarantine of persons with close contacts, guidance to help public understand and adhere to the control measures, prompt effective high-level policy decisions, complete activation of the public health system, full involvement of society – see *Nature*, 2020 (19 August).

On the other hand, on 8 April 2020, the disease in the USA was reaching its peak. All the same, on 14 April 2020, President Trump announced that his country would stop funding the WHO because "(t)he WHO pushed China's misinformation about the virus" and as a result "so much death has been caused by their mistakes." On 2 April 2021, figures from Worldometer (see Table 8.2) showed that in the Total Cases/1 Million population, the USA topped the chart at 94,026, followed by Sweden at 80,145. China showed a figure of 63.

On 30/08/2022, Worldometer released the following figures regarding the countries selected here; Statista on 29/08/2022 released its figures. (In Table 8.1 below, Worldometer figures precede the Statista ones and are in standard font while those provided by Statista are in italics):

Country	Total Cases	Total Deaths	Total Cases/1 M pop	Deaths/I M pop
World	606,930,662	6,491,112	77,864	832.7
USA	96,091,120/ *96,011,855*	1,069,499/*1,069,132*	Not given	Not given
India	44,429,258/ *44,415,723*	[a] Not given/*527,799*	31,527	375
France	34,509,961/ *34,478,797*	154,039/ *153,857*	526, 190	2,349
Brazil	34,397,205/ *34,384,747*	683,718/ *683,548*	159,383	3,168
UK	23,492,875/ *23,492,875*	187,761/ *187,761*	343,191	2,735
S. Korea	23,142.479/ *23,026,960*	26,689/ *26,618*	450,556	520
Russia	19,482,648/ *19,405,923*	384,254/ *384,083*	133,380	2,631
Vietnam	11,408,952	43,117	114,980	435
Australia	10,018.037	13,834	383,284	529
DPRK	4.772.813	74	183,413	3
Belgium	4,484,315	32,516	383,160	2,780
Sweden	2,564,423	19,779	250,556	1,933
Singapore	1,837,090	1,592	308,782	268
Hong Kong	1,531,308	9,683	200,748	1,269
Uruguay	979,160	7,445	279,787	2,127
Egypt	515,645	24,613	4,842	231
Qatar	428,791	681	152,714	243
Kenya	338,170	5,674	6,004	101
Nigeria	263,407	3,148	1,213	14
Zimbabwe	256.704	5,593	16,746	365
China	242,689	5,226	169	4

Table 8.1 Some COVID-19 statistics for selected countries
The death figure at [a] for India is very controversial as there are no agreed official statistics which in turn affect other figures based on it.[3]

[3] The WHO (5 May 2022) holds that many countries undercounted the numbers who died from COVID-19 – for instance, in India there were 4.7 million deaths, 10 times its official figures and almost a third of all such deaths globally. (See Grimley, Cornish and Stylianou 2022; Biswas 2022.) The latest figures (April 2023) show the death toll to be at only 530,901. "…according to the WHO and other scientists and analysts, this is a significant undercount, with officials accused of covering up the

Another set of figures dated earlier (2 April 2021) from Worldometer – see Table 8.2 below – shows that the same ranking between countries has been more or less preserved between the 16 months which had lapsed, although the two Tables serve to show the dynamic nature of the COVID-19 phenomenon. A set of figures can only give a slice of it on any given date – for a full discussion of the changing character of SARS-CoV-2, see WHO, 2022 (11 August).

Date: 2 April 2021	Figures from Worldometer	Total Cases/1 M pop	Deaths/1 M pop
		In Descending Order	In Descending Order
		USA 94, 026 Sweden 80,145 Belgium 76,364 Netherlands 75,026 Spain 70,376 France 71, 810 UK 63,880 Brazil 60,099 Italy 60,088 Germany 34, 056 Japan 3,784 S. Korea 2,031 Hong Kong 1,525 Australia 1,140 New Zealand 500 Thailand 414 Cambodia 151 China 63 Taiwan 44 Vietnam 27	Belgium 1,982 UK 1,861 Italy 1,821 USA 1,705 Spain 1,615 Brazil 1,523 France 1,468 Sweden 1,330 Netherlands 966 Germany 920 Japan 73 Australia 35 S Korea 34 Hong Kong 27 New Zealand 5 China 3 Thailand 1 Cambodia 0.9 Taiwan 0.4 Vietnam 0.4

Table 8.2 Earlier set of figures from Worldometer 2 April 2021

The two Tables show that the highest rate of infection and death occurred in the main in Western countries, led by the two major Anglophone ones, USA and UK but with the exception of Australia and New Zealand situated in the West Pacific region. They also show that the mortality rate is

true extent of the deaths. The WHO estimates that there were about 4,7 m COVID-19 deaths in India by the end of 2021, nearly 10 times more than official records" (Ellis-Petersen 2023).

independent of either a country's raw GDP or PPP (Power Purchasing Parity) – in 2021, the US GDP per capita was 69,288 USD while that of China was 11,188 USD, only a sixth of the US figure. Yet the USA in Table 8.2 stands at the highest level of Total Cases/1 M pop and China is third from the bottom. For Deaths/1 M pop, the USA, according to Table 8.2 stands at the fourth highest position at 4 digits while China appears at the fifth from the bottom at single digit.

The discussion here is severely limited and does not explore why such discrepancies noted above occurred. It is confined to looking in some depth at one particular intervention, namely, mask-wearing, a non-pharmaceutical/Epidemiological measure to control COVID-19. It attempts to show that such measures are embedded within a value-framework which varies from country to country, nation-state to nation-state, culture to culture in different parts of the world. In other words, it is geopolitics at work, taking it beyond a purely medical/scientific context. To put it in another way, it is to show that medicine/Medical Thinking itself is not value-free.

However, the data so far cited are dated April 2021 (Table 8.2) and August 2022 (Table 8.1). One should point out that they reflect, in the case of China, the outcome of pursuing its zero-COVID-19 policy. In December 2022, China altered that policy, abruptly it even appeared, scrapping the use of its primary COVID-19 tracking app, domestic travel restrictions, allowing people with mild or no symptoms to home quarantine as well as permitting from early January 2023 overseas visitors to enter the country without having to go into quarantine. (See *Nature* 9 December 2022; *The Guardian* 29 December 2022.) Is this U-turn plain panic and insanity? It could be explained and understood in the following terms:

(a) China did not lead the pack of countries overturning the zero-COVID-19 policy; as a matter of fact, it followed others such as Australia and New Zealand. (Australia abandoned it by late 2021 and New Zealand finally by September 2022.) Admittedly, these countries have their own unique characteristics which China does not share, such as in terms of the latter's population size and population density.

(b) It must be admitted that the timing was not ideal, being winter, the peak influenza season. However, the Spring Festival/*Chunjie* was in January 2023, the single most significant holiday in the Chinese cultural calendar.[4] Workers from all parts of China make their way back to their distant home village or town for the festivities. Masses of people on the

[4] Traditionally, the celebrations begin on New Year's eve with the family re-union dinner and lasts a total of 16 days. For 2023, this would cover 21 January to 5 February 2023.

move from one end of a large country to the other are a potent factor in the transmission of an infectious disease. Yet, preventing travel for the festival would be hard for the people who had missed seeing their families and their loved ones for such a long time.

(c) Vaccines have become available, even if the home-produced varieties are considered by some to be less effective than those produced in the West. However, it is said that its vaccine policy drive has not been rigorous, leaving some 70% of people aged 60 or older with 40% of those aged 80 or more who might be suffering from vaccine hesitancy exposed to catching the virus.

(d) Businesses, especially small enterprises were facing difficulties in surviving, if not actual bankruptcy during the period of the zero-COVID-19 policy which had been maintained for almost three years. While the health of the nation was/is an important goal of government policy, so was/is the economic health of the country. It had/has to maintain a balance between these two values, being caught between a rock and a hard place. The government was facing protests mounted for such and other reasons listed above. As a matter of fact, the government had intended to modify the zero-COVID-19 policy incrementally following the CPC's 20th Party Congress (16 October – 22 October 2022).

A tragedy then occurred on 24 November 2022 – a fire broke out in an apartment block in Urumqi, Xinjiang which was under strict lockdown, killing ten people. This sparked protests across the country, with many protesters blaming the government's strict COVID-19 regulations for the tragedy, although the local Fire Brigade explained it in terms of its inability to access the block as quickly as possible owing to the narrowness of the road/lane leading to it.

The issues mentioned above led Beijing to lift its zero-COVID-19 policy somewhat suddenly in December 2022 which in turn led to a dramatic increase in confirmed cases of COVID-19 as well as deaths arising from it. Different sources cite different figures; it is difficult to ascertain the veracity of such figures, whatever their provenance.[5] However, here is a set, based on data made available by the WHO, presented via Our World in Data.

---

[5] For one assessment, see Lai and Tatem 2023; for another, see Glanz, Hvistendahl, and Chang, 2023 who published these figures: China's official count is 83,150 deaths as opposed to 1.6 million deaths using a model based on the Shanghai outbreak. The article argued that if the higher estimate is correct or nearer the truth, then this would be embarrassing to the CPC (the ruling Communist Party of China), undermining Xi Jinping's portrayal of China's earlier success as evidence of China's

Date:	Date:	Cumulative Confirmed Cases of Infection	Cumulative Confirmed Cases of Death
		In Descending Order	In Descending Order
10/12/2022		USA 97,600,000 India 44,670,000 China 9,770,000	USA 1,070,000 India 530,653 China 30,884
	26/04/2023	USA 103,080,000 China 99,240,000 India 44,910,000	USA 1, 120, 000 India 531,369 China 120,915

Table.8.3 Figures from Our World in Data on 10 December 2022 and 26 April 2023

These three countries have been selected for the following comments: China and India are more or less equivalent in population if not in geographical size – other things being equal, one would have expected that the cumulative confirmed cases would be roughly the same. Yet the actual figures cited above (26/04/2023) show that India only has less than half the number recorded in China. The anomaly could be explained by the fact that the Indian figures are not reliable – see footnote 3 earlier in the chapter. As for the difference in the figures for the USA and China, one would like to observe that China (in 2020) had 1.44 billion in terms of population which is 4.35 times that of the USA (331 million). Yet, in terms of the number of people affected (26/4/2023), the USA exceeds that of China by slightly over 3 million and in terms of deaths, by around 10 times. If this analysis of the figures is plausible, Beijing can still hold its head up high at least in comparison with what the US government had "achieved", so to speak, in spite of its GDP, its economic might and its hegemonic status in the world. India, which is the world's largest democracy, but comparable in population size with its East Pacific neighbour, nevertheless, shows figures in terms of its cumulative confirmed deaths slightly over 4 times that of China. It is, however, undeniably true that China's figures for cumulative confirmed deaths show a four-fold increase since its abandonment of its zero-COVID-

superiority over the West. See also Chang, South China Morning Post 2023 (4 March) for a report on the outcome of this period of the Spring Festival/Chunjie or the Chinese New Year.

19 policy till recently (that is, between 10 December 2022 and 26 April 2023).

Here is yet another set of data, also from Our World in Data, but based on daily confirmed cases and confirmed deaths which show more clearly how the dramatic increase in confirmed cases and confirmed deaths occurred in China between December 2022 and January 2023 following its abandonment of the zero-COVID-19 policy.

Date	Country	Confirmed Cases	Confirmed Deaths
Dec 19, 2022 April 30, 2023	USA	63,716.29 12, 354.86	378.86 149.43
Dec 20, 2022 April 30. 2023	India	211.43 7,638.57	1.29 29.14
	China		
Dec 8, 2022		21,231.29	47.00
Dec 25, 2022		5,880,000.00	685.00
Dec 30,2022		4,020,000.00	1,494.86
Jan. 2, 2023		2,610,000.00	2,356.14
Jan.9, 2023		872,574,86	3,887.71
Jan.12, 2023		499,208.43	3,373.86
Jan. 29, 2023		22,668.57	502.00
April 30, 2023		440.29	5.14

Table 8.4. Our World in Data: Daily Confirmed Cases and Confirmed Deaths on the Dates Selected

Mask-wearing in COVID-19: Through the Lens of Different Cultural-Ethical/Philosophical Perspectives

It is relevant here to give a brief history of mask-wearing as a public health measure pre- and during COVID-19. In China, where the epidemic was first officially declared to have happened, mask-wearing in Wuhan, the epicentre, became mandatory in January 2020, followed by Shanghai in February 2020. Before COVID-19, mask-wearing was a common phenomenon in China; this was because people chose to wear masks especially in the winter months when colds were widespread or when pollution levels were high. In other areas of East and Southeast Asia, mask-wearing became mandatory also during 2020 – Vietnam on 16 March 2020, Singapore 15 April 2020, South Korea 26 May 2020, Hong Kong 29 July 2020 and Taiwan by December 2020. In Japan, no mandate was issued but just a reminder that one ought to wear masks, given that the habit of mask-wearing was/is very well entrenched. The Hong Kong government, too, could have chosen to issue only a reminder, as people in Hong Kong had taken to wearing masks well before the end of July 2020; however, its government chose to make the matter mandatory.[6]

The WHO in early April 2020 stated that masks must be won not by the public but by front line health workers, people with COVID-19 symptoms as well as carers of infected people. Two months later, in June 2020, its position had altered, stating that the general public should wear face coverings, a guideline it has stuck to since. Furthermore, the WHO also gave instructions to make one's own cloth masks which were said to be effective in the job they were expected to perform.

The WHO and epidemiologists the world over have emphasised that mask-wearing is only one strategy amongst others which society must practise as part of a combination of measures in order to achieve the desired outcome of lowering the infection rate of COVID-19. These other strategies include physical/social distancing, hand washing, not touching one's own face, and even cleaning of public surfaces for fear of what is called fomite transmission (the virus staying on hard surfaces such as handrails, counters, baskets and trolleys in supermarkets after infected people have touched them). However, as medical scientists learned more about the mechanism of transmission, that SARS-CoV-2 transmits primarily by droplets and aerosols, other strategies have been more emphasised which then crucially include mask-wearing, physical/social distancing as well as proper ventilation of indoor spaces.

In England, on 5 July 2021, the government, in the belief that it had successfully rolled out its vaccination programme announced that from 19 July 2021 mask-wearing would no longer be mandatory, but an entirely voluntary affair. However, the Prime Minister almost immediately back-pedalled and changed its language to say that people would, all the same, be "expected" to wear them in crowded indoor areas such as public transport and shops. London for Transport said in response it would continue to demand mask-wearing on its different transport networks; the mayor of Manchester also said that its tram network would continue its mask-wearing policy.

In the USA, on 29 February 2020, the Surgeon General, Dr Jerome Adamas proclaimed on Twitter that masks "are NOT effective in preventing [sic] general public from catching Coronavirus (Cramer and Sheik 2020.)".

---

[6] One should recall that Hong Kong had directly experienced the earlier SARS epidemic of 2003, caused by what today is labelled SARS-CoV-1. The people of Hong Kong, therefore, had taken to mask-wearing well before the SARS-CoV-2/COVID-19 pandemic was officially declared.

The director of the CDC (Center for Disease Control and Prevention), Dr Robert Redfield, in February 2020 also said that healthy people did not need to wear masks although the CDC revised its recommendations on 3 April 2020; and on 14 July 2020, the director in an editorial he co-authored in the *Journal of the American Medical Association* advocated universal masking. He did the same again on 16 September 2020 when he testified before the Senate Appropriations Committee. In March 2020, the director of NIAID (National Institute of Allergy and Infectious Diseases, USA), Dr Anthony Fauci similarly held that mask-wearing might make people feel a little bit better and it might even block a droplet, but it's not providing the perfect protection that people think that it is." He changed his mind later by April 2020. [7]

A study released in June 2021 by the Universities of Bristol, Oxford and Copenhagen analysed the effect of mask-wearing on 20 million people in 92 regions world-wide.[8] It found that mask-wearing by an entire population led to a median reduction in the R number [9] of 25.8% and that the median reduction in R observed in each region in association with mask-wearing was 20.4%. This study establishes the effectiveness of mass mask-wearing and highlights that wearing data, not mandate data, is necessary to infer this effect.[10]

Some governments and officials such as Anthony Fauci of NIAID (USA) chose initially to even prevent mask-wearing as far as the public was concerned for fear that the rush for masks on the part of the public would mean not enough left for front-line health workers. That the richest country in the world had found itself facing a shortage of masks is something of a paradox which, however, can be explained in terms of its philosophy of management which maximises profits and efficiency but at the expense of resilience through outsourcing the production of goods to other economies which could produce them cheaper. As a result, China produces 80% of the world's masks.

---

[7] See "To Mask or Not to Mask? CDC's Mixed Messages During the Pandemic" 2023; "How Masks Went From Don't-Wear to Must-Have 2020"; O'Rourke 2020.

[8] See Leech, Rogers-Smith, Sandbrink, *et al.* 2021.

[9] It is the basic reproduction number, or R_o. It estimates the number of people who will be infected by the average infectious person. It is a critical concept in any attempt at epidemiological modelling.

[10] An earlier publication (De, Goldstein, Morgunov, *et al.* 2020), through its modelling, has argued that near universal masking (80%-90% of the population even with mask efficiency around 70%), in good time (by Day 50 of a pandemic), would have a clear effect in infection mitigation. It is not till early September 2021 that the results of an actual large RCT have become available – for details see footnote 13.

The science behind mask-wearing

In order to develop effective control measures, scientists must investigate the mode of transmission of SARS-CoV-2. Simplistically put, scientists know that respiratory pathogens use two routes, the airborne route and the droplet route, but they did not initially know enough about the relevant variables which governed the actual path taken by a new pathogen such as SARS-CoV-2. Droplets are larger particles than aerosols; in the droplet-borne route, the disease is transmitted by large droplets (> 100 μm) or medium droplets (between 5 and 100 μm) which fall to the ground or land on other surfaces soon after release because of gravity – this is also called the fomite route (hence hand washing, cleaning surfaces such as counters, supermarket trolleys, using hand sanitisers are said to be relevant measures to obstruct this route of transmission). Should the virus predominantly take the airborne route, the disease is transmitted by aerosols and small droplets (< 5 μm) which can be short-distance or longer-range. However, the scientific consensus up to the end of May 2020 as seen in this overview (Hooper 2020 published by the Massachusetts General Hospital) is that "there is strong evidence from the SARS epidemic… and the current COVID-19 pandemic … to suggest that this virus is predominantly transmitted via the droplet and contact routes. There is no evidence that SARS-CoV-2 is an obligate or a preferential aerosol-transmitted airborne disease in the community…" The scientific community, at any one moment in time, was necessarily ignorant about all the relevant aspects of the nature of the new coronavirus and its mode of operation. This a very important point to bear in mind.

There are masks and masks but the broadest two main types will first be distinguished – those worn by front-line health workers who have the closest contact with people with very serious or serious infection of COVID-19 and those worn by the rest of the general public who may be asymptomatic or presymptomatic but who are, nevertheless, capable of infecting others with COVID-19.

The former category (worn in the main by professionals) are respirator masks called FFP ("filtering face pieces"). What do they filter? They filter or keep out salt and oil particles – hence they can be of a variety of sizes and fittings, ranging from FFP1 which can keep out 80%, FFP2 94% and FFP3 99% of such particles. Such high efficiency in filtering brings in its wake a problem – the wearer of such a type of mask finds it difficult to breathe while wearing it. Hence, a valve may be designed in its construction which then suffers from the drawback of allowing some unfiltered out-going air from the wearer to escape, which may go on to infect some other person in the vicinity of the wearer. Whatever the anomalies, this is the only type appropriate for use in a clinical setting. They do the job of protecting the wearer of the mask from being infected by those people who are already infected with COVID-19 (that is, the patients) whom the clinical staff have to treat. So ironically there arises a situation where the person wearing such a type of mask may turn out to be an agent in infecting others – for this reason, the California Bay Area had banned the wearing of such masks with valves in public. However, in the clinical situation, to prevent such a consequence from happening, staff who wear PPFs also wear a shield – such a combination serves to protect the health worker as well as the patient.

In principle one could argue that in epidemiological terms, it makes sense for everyone, whether clinical or ordinary member of the public to wear PPFs. In practice, this policy is defective for several reasons: respirator masks plus shield would be cumbersome for everyone to use, the combination would be costly, and worst of all, demand may exceed supply when the greatest fear would arise, namely, that front-line health workers would be left bereft of the equipment.

As epidemiological strategy, the public in general are either mandated or strongly encouraged to wear not respirator masks but disposable masks (the material commonly used is polypropylene) which are generally flat and pleated with a built-in nose wire and simple elastic straps that go around the ears. Or they are cloth masks, with more than one layer of fabric. The primary function of such masks is simply to prevent the exhaled breath of the wearer from reaching other people – as people can be asymptomatic or presymptomatic, wearing such a mask would trap the droplets which may contain the coronavirus from travelling further afield. [11]

In summary, one could say that respirator (PPF) masks used in clinical settings primarily protect the wearers from infection while the masks worn by the public serve primarily to prevent spreading the wearers' own germs to others rather than to protect them from being infected by those around

[11] This is called "source control". Research has shown that the average human cough fills roughly three quarters of a two-litre soda bottle with air which shoots out of the lungs in a jet. Also, each cough releases as many as 3000 droplets of saliva at speeds of up to 50 miles per hour. The sneeze starts from the back of the throat and exudes even more droplets, as many as 40,000 some of which gush out at speeds greater than 200 miles per hour. These droplets are so tiny, less than 100 microns across, that we cannot see them with our naked eye. The larger droplets fall to the ground quite quickly because of the force of gravity. The smaller and lighter ones (five microns or less) are not affected by gravity and can stay afloat for a good long while if not almost indefinitely in a room with little or no adequate air flow. Once airborne, viruses in the tiny droplets can survive for hours.

them. However, studies have also shown that such masks (which may be called ordinary masks) worn by the public do provide a degree of protection to the wearers of the mask (the mask absorption rate).[12] The chopping and changing of views regarding the efficacy of masks in reducing transmission of the virus was settled when the results of a very large RCT were announced. [13]

---

[12] The Mayo Clinic Staff 2021 writes: "A cloth mask is intended to trap respiratory droplets that are released when the wearer talks, coughs or sneezes. **It also acts as a barrier to protect the wearer from inhaling droplets released by others**. The most effective cloth masks are made of multiple layers of tightly woven fabric like cotton. A mask with layers will stop more droplets from getting through your mask or escaping from it."

Maragakis 2021 (John Hopkins Medicine) writes: "If you are infected with the coronavirus and do not know it, a mask is very good at keeping your respiratory droplets and particles from infecting others. If you haven't yet received your COVID-19 vaccine, **wearing a mask can also help prevent germs that come from another person's respiratory droplets from getting into your nose and mouth.**" The CDC, USA on 7 May 2021 writes in similar vein: "SARS-CoV-2 infection is transmitted predominately by inhalation of respiratory droplets generated when people cough, sneeze, sing, talk, or breathe. CDC recommends community use of masks, specifically non-valved multi-layer cloth masks, to prevent transmission of SARS-CoV-2. Masks are primarily intended to reduce the emission of virus-laden droplets ("source control"), which is especially relevant for asymptomatic or presymptomatic infected wearers who feel well and may be unaware of their infectiousness to others, and who are estimated to account for more than 50% of transmissions. Masks also help reduce inhalation of these droplets by the wearer ("filtration for wearer protection"). The community benefit of masking for SARS-CoV-2 control is due to the combination of these effects; individual prevention benefit increases with increasing numbers of people using masks consistently and correctly."

[13] See Chow 2021 about a major RCT recently completed in Bangladesh involving more than 340,000 people across 600 villages to investigate what effect mask wearing may have on COVID -19 infection. The study reports "an 11.9 percent decrease in symptomatic Covid symptoms and a 9.3 percent reduction in symptomatic seroprevalence, which indicates that the virus was detected in blood tests." One of the researchers of the project is also reported as having said: "A 30-percent increase in mask-wearing led to a 10 percent drop in Covid, so imagine if there was a 100-percent increase – if everybody wore a mask and we saw a 100-percent change." However, this kind of large-scale RCT is not often practical and therefore, readily achievable; furthermore, it takes time to complete, and time is a scarce commodity in epidemiological terms when an infectious disease is growing exponentially – see Greenhaigh 2021.

Different cultures perceive mask-wearing in different moral, cultural light: Low Individualism and High Individualism[14]

Putting things simplistically, let us use the USA, on the one hand, to stand for the extreme end of a spectrum (High Individualism/HI) and East Asian countries (China, Japan, Thailand, Vietnam and so forth) to stand at the other end (Low Individualism/LI). The USA is made to represent the Western moral-social-cultural paradigm and East Asian countries are made to represent, in contrast, an expression of the non-Western moral-social-cultural paradigm.[15]

In the USA, in spite of a higher declared intention to wear masks amongst the population, mask-wearing resistance was not insignificant, manifested noisily not only in terms of actual protests and demonstrations but also in the language resisters used, a language which embodied and manifested their ideological worldview, declaring that the epidemiological measure constituted a violation of their Constitutional rights. [16] In contrast, the UK protesters were more muted in the numbers who turned up to protest. In what should have been a high-profile, media-attracting demonstration in

---

[14] It is important to point out that the issue of mask-wearing should not be discussed in a context-free manner. For instance, wearing masks in a heavily air polluted environment is very different from wearing them during an epidemic/pandemic. In the former context, the wearers are simply protecting the self from harm without any possibility of preventing similar harm to others; in the latter context, the wearers are primarily protecting others although mask wearing may to some extent also benefit the self. From the moral standpoint, the two contexts are very different.

[15] It is not about the actual statistics of mask-wearing in these countries or the declaration of intent to wear one on the part of those polled in these countries. For instance, according to the BBC 2020 (July 20), Americans had generally accepted mask-wearing more readily than people in the UK – nearly 60% in the US said they would always wear a mask when they went outside compared to less than 20% in the UK. Table 8.3 in the text makes the same point. In other words, what is explored in some detail is how different cultures perceive the epidemiological measure of mask-wearing in general, and in particular, how different cultures either justify it or justify rejecting it.

[16] In Minnesota, 36 parent groups representing more than 30,0000 families wrote to the State Governor Tim Walz as well as President Joe Biden saying they "have watched the last week unfold in abject horror," referring to schools calling for mandatory mask-wearing. They used language as follows: "We are here to inform you that your uninvited reign of destruction over the children of Minnesota is finished". The children "are ours, and they, too, are Americans with rights". Other groups in Minnesota also signed the open letter – see Williams 2021.

London when masks were made mandatory, only about a mere 100 or so gathered in Hyde Park. Furthermore, they did not cite the Magna Carta or similar highfalutin political rhetoric (Sky News UK, 2020). They simply said that the legislation would infringe civil liberties and that it was not supported by the Science, so to speak. They maintained that there was no scientific consensus about the benefits of wearing masks, that the WHO had changed their minds several times, and so had the CDC, USA. Their message was "spread love not fear". [17] (See also Figure 8.1 below.)

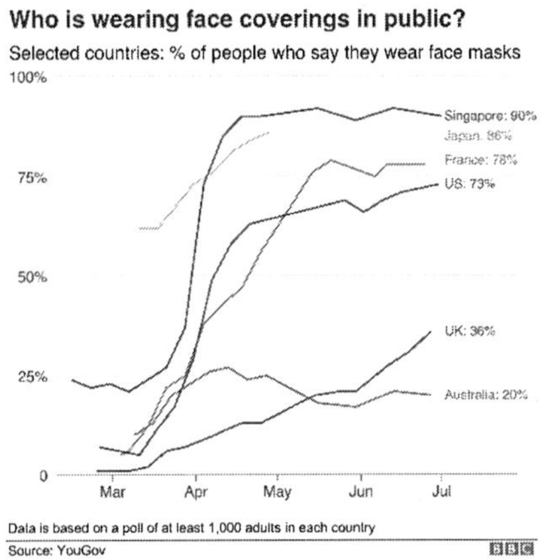

Figure 8.1

On yet another obvious level, among the resisters in the USA there appeared to be more supporters and voters of the Republican Party than the Democratic Party – a Gallup poll found that nearly 100% of Democrats polled wore a mask when going out compared to 70% of Republicans, a gap which had increased since the last poll three months earlier (see Hogberg 2020). This is unsurprising. Trump, as President of the USA at the time when the pandemic hit his country, had dismissed the threat posed by the

[17] What they said was true then. However, there is a need to bear in mind one important thing about how Science and scientists work – the scientific procedure is a dynamic one, as already observed. In some areas, the rate of change in the understanding and perception of a phenomenon is so fast that a few weeks or months might make a lot of difference, especially in a domain where little is known beforehand, such as when a new coronavirus like SARS-CoV-2 gets a hold in a country. Science is a collective effort, involving researchers and practitioners in all relevant domains of knowledge such as physics, chemistry, biology, medicine, sociology, anthropology, psychology, technology especially in big data computer technology, not to mention even philosophy.

virus, claiming that everything was under control even as cases continued to increase. He then blamed the media and the Democrats in these words on 9/03/2020: "The Fake New Media and their partner, the Democrat Party, is doing everything within its semi-considerable power (it used to be greater!) to inflame the CoronaVirus (sic) situation far beyond what the facts would warrant. Surgeon General, 'The risk is low to the average American'."

On 13/03/2020, Trump declared a national emergency, insisting that he had not shifted his position and that "I've always known this is a real, this is a pandemic. (sic) I've felt it was a pandemic long before it was called a pandemic." Yet, on 29/05/2021, he withdrew the USA from the WHO on the grounds that China had "pressured the World Health Organization to mislead the world when the virus was first discovered by Chinese authorities." However, by late July, his tone had moved up another sombre gear, this time to get the nation to wear masks, although he had downplayed mask-wearing up to then; indeed, he had mocked Biden earlier for wearing one. For the first time in public, at least, he wore a mask on 12/07/2020 against a background of rising cases of infection (66, 528 infections over 24 hours) and death (a total of almost 135,000 deaths since the pandemic had taken off). On 02/10/2020, Trump and his wife tested positive for the virus. That same night he was transferred by helicopter to the Walter Reed Medical Center. On 05/10/2020, he discharged himself from hospital to continue his presidential campaign trail, against all known COVID-19 protocols. And so, he continued in such a vein even after he lost the election (early November 2020) to Biden.[18]

Perhaps it would be more correct to call the USA phenomenon the Trump Phenomenon. The Trump Phenomenon may be analysed in terms of several interrelated elements. First, underlying it is the minimal view of the state, associated with von Hayek's *The Road to Serfdom*, 1944 which argued that an appropriate system of government should leave individuals to pursue what they perceive to be their self-interest with the minimum direction from above, as that is the best system for managing uncertainty and change. The market, for instance, exemplifies best this kind of arrangement at work – vendors sell what they want to sell and at the price determined by what buyers are willing to pay. Both buyers and sellers get mutual satisfaction though each is acting entirely from the standpoint of self-interest – a spontaneous order appears even though no obvious hand is directing it. One

[18] BBC, 2020 (July 12); Greenberg and Sherman 2021.

could see Hayek as a successor to Adam Smith's hidden hand of the market.[19]

However, this is not to say that the majority of mask-wearing "refusniks" would know anything about the minimal state. It is to say that the minimal state view has entered their blood stream, and therefore informed their thinking and their conduct without their knowing it. [20] As a result, they said that mandatory mask-wearing constitutes a violation of their liberties which include the right to make choices about one's health and bodily integrity, that individuals can choose to allow themselves to be infected by the coronavirus spewed out by others should they so wish, just as one may drink as much alcohol as one wants, that any interference from the state with one's choice is, therefore, unjustified and is a manifestation of the nanny or paternalistic state. Furthermore, they would regard mandatory mask-wearing as violation of the First Amendment right to assembly and association.[21] Vice President Mike Pence said: "I want to remind you again freedom of speech and the right to peaceably assemble is in the Constitution of the U.S. Even in a health crisis, the American people don't forfeit our constitutional rights." [22]

Second, the minimal view of the state is associated with Individualism as an ideological worldview. The USA in general is perceived to embody

---

[19] However, some theorists consider Hayek was, at best, a moderate libertarian and argue that the true founder of the minimal state is Robert Nozick (*Anarchy, State, and Utopia, 1*974). His minimal state possesses two main attributes or performs two functions: monopoly or near monopoly of force in the territory as well as protective or security services for everyone within the territory. When a state goes beyond these two tasks, then rights will be violated.

[20] Philosophers, following Merleau-Ponty, have called this process of the cultural absorption of philosophical worldviews *sédimentation.* Baggini, 2018, xiii-xiv: "Most people do not consciously articulate the philosophical assumptions they have absorbed and are often not even aware that they have any, but assumptions about the nature of self, ethics, sources of knowledge, the goals of life, are deeply embedded in our cultures and frame our thinking without our being aware of them."

[21] Unlike the concept of the minimal state which forms part of the US *sédimentation,* the USA Constitution is always at the forefront of American consciousness.

[22] Pence has been shown to be wrong: the First Amendment is not absolute, though ensured by the Constitution. The US Supreme Court has long recognised that protecting public health is a legitimate end which can override measures that might otherwise violate the First Amendment or other provisions in the Bill of Rights. (See Finn 2020; Fink 2020.) A case brought to court in Minnesota on such grounds was rejected by the judge who considered the argument "meritless". Other resisters used "My body, My Choice", re-cycled from feminist campaigners against those who wish to ban abortion especially on religious ground.

the spirit of Individualism and in that sense to be the leading nation in the world in a list of individualist nations and cultures. Others perceived to belong to that tradition but with decreasing stridency are Australia, UK, Netherlands, New Zealand. [23] The term and concept of Individualism is somewhat slippery and one must define it for the purpose of the discussion here. It is used in the following senses. It is not used here in opposition to what is normally called Collectivism. [24] Instead, a spectrum is invoked with High Individualism/HI at one end and Low Individualism/LI at the other. To reframe: one could say that the USA stands at the high end of Individualism. High Individualism focuses on the individual as a self-contained entity or as a free-floating social atom and considers society to be no more than a mere collection of such social atoms with no cohesive or adhesive bonds between them (apart possibly from the immediate family of the individual) and so can, without remainder, be reduced to the sum of these social atoms.

High Individualism appears, at first sight, to have affinity with Classical Liberalism via John Stuart Mill's distinction between self-regarding and other-regarding acts. However, the affinity disappears upon closer inspection. Mill was content to say that as the category of self-regarding acts covered those which harmed only the individual though it might annoy or irritate others, the individual should be left well alone to perform them. High Individualism appears in certain contexts such as mask-wearing to go beyond Mill by appearing to eliminate the category of the other-regarding acts which individuals, according to Mill, are not permitted to do since they cause harm to others. So, while Mill recognised duties to others, High Individualists appear to elide the distinction. For them, it looks as if individuals have the right to do whatever they want or desire to do *carte blanche*, irrespective of damaging consequences their actions may cause to others. Such libertarians are, therefore, not liberals in the classical understanding of Liberalism. The preferred language of High Individualism

[23] See Hofstede n.d. Although Canada does not appear as a separate entry, it is generally assumed that it stands shoulder-to-shoulder with the USA along this spectrum.

[24] The term "Collectivism" is best avoided as it is often associated with terms such as "totalitarianism", "authoritarianism"; such terms imply concepts which not only leave no room for moral agency on the part of individual persons but also that they are only capable of having orders imposed upon them from above. The approach here avoids the normal distinction between Individualism and Collectivism. Instead, it postulates High Individualism at one end of the Individualism spectrum and Low Individualism at the other end. However, Hofstede (end of 1970s) retained the Individualism-Collectivism distinction in his model of national cultures.

is that of rights, human rights, fundamental rights, constitutional rights, interpreted in absolutist terms, eschewing the language of duties and responsibilities to others. When disagreements and conflicts emerge between individuals, High Individualism resorts either to the use of military might (not perhaps so much in the domestic but not infrequently in the international/geopolitical context); in the domestic context, it typically resorts to litigation, lawsuits and the courts to settle disputes.

In contrast, nations and cultures towards the Low Individualism end of the spectrum recognise that apart from the rights of individuals, there are also responsibilities and duties to others. The People's Republic of China may be considered to stand at the extreme Low Individualism end of the spectrum with Singapore, Thailand, South Korea, Taiwan and Hong Kong closely following behind. In other words, there are moral, social, cultural bonds between individuals which make society possible as a structured, coherent whole. In the evolutionary history of humankind, initially the meaningful unit of society was the family and the tribe, then groups of tribes or clans in a specific region, next the merging of these to become a larger whole with an overall jurisprudential authority in charge which one call the state, and finally in recent modern times, they even see themselves as a nation-state.

Low Individualism also necessarily emphasises harmony and co-operation as central values as, in their absence, society could well fracture and disintegrate. As a moral/social/political/cultural concept, harmony crucially recognises that while disagreements and conflicts between individuals/groups will always exist, nevertheless, they have to be peacefully resolved if society, the Whole, is to continue to exist and to flourish. Paradoxically, they imply adherence to Mill's two categories of duties although it is correct to observe that their category of the other-regarding acts may be larger in terms of membership of such acts than in their category of the self-regarding acts. However, they are not the mirror image of Libertarianism under High Individualism, as they do not elide the distinction; only they tend to endorse more acts coming under the other-regarding than they do under the self-regarding category.

It follows then that Low Individualism is not compatible with the philosophy of the minimal state. To put the matter a little differently, one could say that while High Individualism regards government or state intervention necessarily to be evil and to be resisted as much as it is possible or even at all cost (to mount revolts and rebellions or so-called "colour revolutions" in today's geopolitical discourse), Low Individualism regards government or state intervention to be both necessary and, therefore, virtuous in principle. [25]

In general, to conclude this section, one could explain why (a) mask-wearing resistance would occur in the most strident form in the USA as it occupies the extreme end of the spectrum as High Individualism; (b) the resistance would be conducted in a language which invokes freedom and autonomy of the individual; (c) mandatory mask-wearing is seen as a violation of the right of the individual which precludes incursion into the personal, sacrosanct space of individuals, of preserving their own health and bodily integrity as they see fit, the outcome entirely of their own decision-making, irrespective fundamentally of causing harm to others or indeed even harm to themselves; (d) typically resisters claimed that it is, above all, a violation of their Constitutional rights under the First Amendment, the most sacred of all rights under their understanding of freedom and democracy. Overall, their ideological worldview is consonant with the view

---

[25] The operative word, here, is "in principle". It is important to point out straight-away that Low Individualism as political philosophy is not committed to endorsing any and every state intervention/government as virtuous, as there are also other values in their philosophical framework to distinguish between good governance and bad governance. If China is taken to stand at the extreme Low Individualism end of the spectrum, one could cite the edicts of bad kings/emperors in its past as exemplars of bad governance. Edicts which decreed that the peasants be "conscripts" in the battles and wars they fought against other rulers and states to augment their own territories and their power in order to achieve hegemonic status, that the peasants be taxed so highly that they and their families could barely survive without getting into debt. Such bad rulers also neglected to maintain existing infrastructures such as rivers and canals for the purpose of efficient irrigation and transportation, to undertake new ones as society developed, who encouraged or failed to stamp out corruption and so forth. Good governance would consist of edicts which permitted the peasants to cultivate their land in peace and security, which did not burden them with crippling taxes, but which helped them to improve their yield of extant crops, to grow new ones and which ultimately meant they lived without corrupt officials, rapacious landlords and so forth. In other words, a good emperor/ ruler was defined in a nutshell as someone who had the welfare of the common people at the heart of their policies. The *dao*/path of good governance consisted of promoting the well-being of the people which was understood to refer fundamentally to their desire for prosperity and security, in the largest sense of the term – no wars ravaging the land, no armies trampling over cultivated fields, no bearing of arms for kings and landlords, no drought, no floods, no famine, no plagues, no political and social disorder, no crippling taxes. This list might consist of well-being only negatively conceived (what is sometimes called negative utilitarianism) but if attained would, in practice, be equivalent to Bentham's principle of the greatest happiness of the greatest number.

of the minimal state and of Libertarianism. However, it is not consonant with Classical Liberalism.

In contrast, countries and cultures towards the Low Individualism end of the spectrum tend to accept mandatory mask-wearing as an edict of the state which is in keeping with their understanding of good governance as well as with their recognition that morally compelling reasons dictate restraint be placed on conduct of the self in order to promote overwhelming benefits to others. Their moral framework accommodates both duties to self and duties to others, and furthermore recognises that given the kind of world we humans live in, there may be more issues and matters falling into the latter category than High Individualism would care to admit.

Exploring further the relation between Self and Others

This section will examine this theme under two aspects, to show that empirically and conceptually the notion of the self is meaningless without reference to others; that these links, together with other features already explored in the section above, would mean that even if mask-wearing only prevents harm to others with no accompanying possibility of preventing harm to self, people in Low Individualism societies/cultures would accept/conform to mask-wearing readily on moral and cultural grounds. On the other hand, it would argue that if mask-wearing exclusively or primarily benefits only others but not the mask-wearer, persons in High Individualism cultures and countries would not consider it morally compelling to wear masks and to resist/reject wearing them.

High Individualism implies that it makes sense to conceptualise the self but to ignore the concept of others, This, to Low Individualism, is philosophically unintelligible. In the largest understanding of language and the reality which language points to beyond itself, the world cannot simply contain the individual, the self in the absence of others. Minimally, it consists of two others – human reproduction (which is sexual reproduction) involves three people, the self and its biological parents. Although it is the female self which carries the child to term, the female self cannot be pregnant without the male other (which has now been expanded through the influx of new technologies). The result of such a pregnancy is yet another other. In other words, for humankind to maintain itself as a species over time, the species must reproduce itself, and this involves minimally four individuals or to put the matter differently, the self and, strange as it may seem at first sight, not even only two but in fact, three others. [26] This then is the logic and arithmetic of human sexual reproduction.

Furthermore, a human infant, unlike other mammalian infants requires intensive nurturing and concerted use of parental-societal resources for healthy growth and development. For a start, humans, given their type of consciousness, have a language which is capable of extreme abstraction; it is this in-built capability for abstraction which enables humans to do sums, to speculate whether God exists, to put forward theories about the motions of the planets. The human infant must be taught language by many others, immediate parents, older siblings, other relatives, neighbours, teachers in schools.

Conceptually, our human language is learnt and transmitted in a manner which involves polar contrasts. Think of terms such as "this", "here", "up", "now", "hot", "light", "day" and so forth. On every occasion of their use, we imply that each term has its own polar contrast within the context it is invoked.

Term	*Polar Contrast*	*Term*	*Polar Contrast*
this	that	day	night
here	there	woman	man
up	down	plant	animal
now	then	grief	joy
hot	cold	birth	death
light	dark	Hell	Heaven

It follows that the term "self" has as its polar contrast the term "other". If our language necessarily embodies the two terms, then it also follows that the two terms stand for two different though related concepts. The

[26] The reasoning is quite obvious. If reproduction requires two individuals but if any two individuals are not having two children, but say only one, then the couple is not reproducing itself. Take this example from the class of 1927 Harvard graduates. This highly educated class according to one set of statistics was committing suicide. The Population Reference Bureau in 1952 showed that the average alumnus of the Class of '27 produced only 1.85 children since graduation – this figure was based on more than 10,000 reports from members of this Class throughout America. The Bureau estimated that 2.1 children were needed for replacement. If the findings of this sample report turned out to be reliable, then extrapolation would show that the 103, 000 individuals who graduated from Harvard that year would bequeath only 79,000 children. If this figure in turn turned out to be correct, then the male graduates of 1927 would have failed to reproduce themselves by 12 per cent. And if this 12 per cent reduction were to persist, then this would ultimately lead to the extinction of the Class of '27. (T*he Harvard Crimson*, 1952 (June 17)).

individual person, the self, in daily existence must know how to negotiate its relationship with others, whether these be one's parents, one's children, one's neighbours, one's friends, the local shop keeper, the local police officer on the beat and so forth. The range of others extends to include one's compatriots, people living in neighbouring countries to all peoples in the world. As the range of relationships with others extends outwards, the self must learn to relate to these others politically, morally and culturally.

High Individualism and Low Individualism understand these relationships with others differently from the moral vantage point. The former's moral boundaries are very tightly drawn as it wants as much as possible to exclude the other/s; the latter draws such boundaries in a more expansive manner, to include as many others in a specific context as it is practical to do. In the context of mask-wearing, the differences in a nutshell pan out as shown in Table 8.5 in the section to follow.

There is yet another way of making the same point, a way indicated by Ingold, 2016. [27] If one had not misunderstood Ingold, a key theme of his extended nuanced exposition seems to be that we, human beings, are par excellence "'an animal which responds' … As responsive beings, the responsibility of care is something that *falls* to us. The actions we carry out in its fulfilment are therefore in the nature of tasks. A task is an action that we owe rather than own: it belongs to others rather than ourselves…". Altering Ingold's language slightly, one could say that Low Individualism embodies and manifests responsivity and responsibility, a moral vantage point which is totally alien to High Individualism, as it ignores or denies the basic premise that humans are "an animal which responds" and which, therefore, makes the human animal a responsible being.

Conclusion

If the arguments advanced in this exploration are empirically plausible and coherently presented, they would have established the following theses:

1 Epidemiology in general and mask-wearing and lockdown as specific public health, non-pharmaceutical measures are best understood within a moral-political-cultural framework which recognises John Stuart Mill's distinction between self-regarding and other-regarding Acts.

Low Individualism cultural frameworks are consonant with above, while High Individualism frameworks with their moral boundaries being tightly drawn around the self-interested individual are not consonant

[27] With thanks to David Ing for drawing attention to it.

with either Classical Liberalism or Epidemiological Thinking and theorising.

2 Epidemiological Thinking characteristically and necessarily situates the self in relation to the other/s in a reciprocal manner such that what benefits/damages others would benefit/damage the self and what benefits/damages the self would benefit/damage others.

One needs here to recognise that Epidemiological Thinking distinguishes between two different contexts in which benefits or damage can occur in a reciprocal manner. The first is when wearing a mask on the part of the wearer (the self) benefits other people around as the mask traps droplets emitted from the self's breath, coughs and sneezes, preventing them from escaping when they could be carrying the coronavirus, SARS-CoV-2. At the same time, wearing the mask could prevent the mask-wearer (the self) from being infected by the disease-bearing droplets, big and small, emitted by others around the self. The second is when even if it turns out that no evidence exists which shows that the mask worn by the self/the mask-wearer protects against droplets containing SARS-CoV-2 emitted by others around the self, Epidemiological Thinking demonstrates that if mask-wearing in a population is near universal (say around 80%), this means that there is less of the pathogen flying about to cause mischief and damage. In other words, the self would still enjoy a much better level of protection from harm when mask-wearing is near universal in the community than when it is not. In this epidemiologically extended manner, wearing a mask to protect others from harm can and does indeed protect the self from harm.[28]

These points made above are encapsulated in Table 8.5 set out below. (However, exploring them in fuller detail will be left to Chapter 9 which examines the concept of Wholism.) Before turning to this task, one should make one other point: mask-wearing is an important Epidemiological strategy in controlling COVID-19, but let us not forget that it is one of a range of non-pharmaceutical measures adopted by countries in the world

---

[28] There are various models in Epidemiology called compartmental models for disease transmission in contagious epidemics. A classic contribution, much cited, is that of Kermack and McKendrick, 1927 which postulated three compartments, the **S**(usceptible) **I** (nfected) **R**(ecovered/emoved through death), the SIR Model. All models make assumptions. This one assumes that initially all members of the community are equally susceptible to the pathogen and that a single infection bestows complete immunity. They performed a mathematical investigation of such a model. Another model called the SEIR Model has four compartments, the additional is **E**(xposed).

and that another significant component of this package of stratagems include the more radical lockdown, a measure which has attracted the maximum of condemnation and wrath on the part of the USA which leads countries positioned at the High Individualism end of the spectrum. The country which receives such denunciation most forcefully is therefore China, which has invoked the lockdown strategy, and stands at the Low Individualism end of the spectrum. Such counties would justify lockdowns in much the same way as they would justify mask-wearing, namely, on the grounds, that while highly inconvenient to the self, on the one hand, but benefitting others, the outcome, however, is also a win-win situation. This is because, on the other hand, in protecting others, one is also at the same time protecting oneself from harm. Medical data appear to bear out this justification – refer to the figures cited for death in Tables 8.1 and 8.2.

Table 8.5 (below) refers to the concepts of Coloniality and Decoloniality. Although one is deferring till the next chapter an exploration of the concept of Low Individualism/LI from the vantage point of Wholism, one needs, straightaway, to provide a gloss on the introduction of these two concepts as follows:

Coloniality in this context refers to the hegemonic power in the world, imposing on other cultural traditions its own epistemological standard while denouncing and down-grading other knowledge-systems as substandard or inferior. Historically, the seat of hegemonic power in the world had been Western Europe since its rise in the seventeenth century, with first England leading the way, followed by France and other European nation-states. This situation lasted for about two centuries until the rise of the USA at the end of WWll to accept that baton of high global status and power. Decoloniality in this context refers to the refusal to accept such hegemonic imposition on the part of the hegemonic power by asserting their own epistemological yardstick.[29]

However, Decoloniality in the context of mask-wearing is not to be understood in the following way: namely, if one were to interview mask-wearers in LI societies and ask why they are wearing masks, the term and concept of Decoloniality would not come tripping merrily off their tongues. Instead, they would probably say it is just common morality or even common sense to do what one can to stop or at least decrease the spread of the virus in the community. However, if they are informed members of the

[29] For a detailed exploration of these two concepts, see Mignolo 2017. (These important geopolitical aspects of knowledge in the world of today, unfortunately, have been overlooked by the well-known evolutionary biologist, Andreas Wagner 2023, in his latest account of the cultural evolution of *Homo Sapiens*.)

public about how other people in other societies and countries are reacting to the virus, they would be aware of the difference in moral/political responses between themselves and those belonging to another cultural tradition, and of the fact that the government of the USA (at least under Trump) was claiming the high moral/geopolitical ground in denouncing the evil government of the Peoples' Republic of China in pursuing epidemiological measures such as lockdown and mask-wearing. Other East Pacific countries like Japan and S. Korea which belong to the tradition of LI (because of their common Confucian value-system) do not see fit to join the USA in denouncing the PRC, even in the case of Japan which in other issues tend to toe the US line. On the issue of mask-wearing in the context of the COVID-19 pandemic, Japan, S. Korea, Singapore have distanced themselves from the stance advocated by the White House. Their conduct, as such, could be understood as tantamount to Decoloniality, albeit a low-profile expression without political shouting and flag-waving. Nonetheless, it constitutes a convincing manifestation of not being a "vassal" state of the USA and its hegemonic stance in the world of geopolitics.

In any case, judging by the data available, it bears repeating that one could plausibly argue that the Chinese efforts and strategies for fighting COVID-19 have produced better outcomes (in terms of confirmed deaths) than those countries (such as the USA) with their different strategies pursued within their own cultural framework. In that sense, the Chinese model of controlling the epidemic/pandemic may be said to be superior. The Chinese model draws upon its underlying cultural tendencies, occupying the Low Individualism end of the spectrum, its moral predisposition to act to promote the value of the common good even at the expense of the self, a value it shares with other East Pacific countries as members of their common Confucian heritage, including a greater reliance on Epidemiological measures rather than Clinical Medical interventions Admittedly, the situation changed dramatically when China, quite suddenly dropped its zero-COVID-19 policy since December 2022, data for confirmed cases of infection and confirmed deaths rose. However, as Table 8.4 shows, within roughly four months, the figures by April 30, 2023, indicate that the virus was under control again – one ought to admit it is an impressive performance.

High Individualism (HI)	Low Individualism (LI)
HI entails a hierarchy of positions, arranged in a descending order below: Should masks protect only the self, reject mask-wearing as the self, given Autonomy and Freedom, may choose to do whatever it wants to do, including the freedom and therefore the right to be infected. Freedom and Autonomy are prioritised even over harm to the self. Call this the Masochistic Version of HI. If masks only protect others but do not protect the self from infection, reject mask-wearing. Call this the self-interested version. If, however, mask-wearing does to an extent also protect the self while over-whelmingly protects others from infection, then the self could/might entertain mask-wearing. This implication follows from the premise of the self as a self-interested individual who seeks to prevent harm to itself – the self would only act if the interests of itself are involved, but not otherwise. Empirical evidence regarding mask-wearing to protect the self from infection does seem to an extent to exist – if this is correct, then mask-wearing resisters ought to revise their stance. Whether they would do so, depends on how highly they price the value of preventing harm to the self. An extreme masochistic version would not value it – in the name of Autonomy and Freedom, it may choose to reject mask-wearing.	Should masks only protect others but do not protect the self from infection, then the self would still mask, as a fundamental value of LI is to avoid causing harm to others through the action of the self. The commitment to mask-wearing to prevent others from infection is reinforced by the fact that the action of mask-wearing involves only a limited degree of inconvenience to the wearer. On the cost-benefit sheet of LI, the cost to the mask-wearer in terms of limited inconvenience is undisputedly out-weighed by the amount of benefit which flows to others through mask-wearing. LI needs only pose this simple question to the self: does the self have a moral duty to wear a mask if mask-wearing on the part of the self would contribute to preventing others from infection? The answer to this question is an unequivocal "Yes." So, such a self would wear a mask. In a society where LI prevails, such a society would achieve the desirable goal of a tolerable low level of infection even if this moral strategy cannot secure a zero rate of infection. If epidemiological evidence shows that masks also to an extent protect the self, then the low rate of infection in the community/society would be reinforced. LI recognises that by acting to bring about a common good – that is, to prevent or decrease the incidence of infection overall in the community/ society – the self in turn can enjoy the good of avoiding infection, as the smaller the number of infected people there is, the less is the chance of the self catching the infection. In other words, LI is a win-win, not a zero-sum game. In

HI in either version is not consonant with Epidemiological reasoning and understanding of SARS-CoV-2/ COVID -19. HI is not consonant with Classical Liberalism. HI denies or ignores the premise that human beings are responsive and therefore, responsible beings. HI obtains in Anglophone countries led by the USA which since the end of WWII and the dissolution of the Soviet Union has assumed the role of imposing Coloniality on other countries using both its hard and soft power. Resistance against mask-wearing constitutes its use of soft power. The UK which usually backs the USA is subdued in the context of mask-wearing.	benefitting others, the self also benefits itself. The paradox of LI: there is no need to make mask-wearing mandatory, although some countries with LI resort to the law (a) to take care of residual cases of recalcitrance and (b) to remind the people that not only is mask-wearing morally compelling but also legally compelling – see Cheng *et al.* 2020, Nakayachi *et al.* 2020. LI, with its built-in concepts of altruism and solidarity is consonant with Epidemiological reasoning and understanding of SARS-CoV-2/COVID-19. LI is consonant with Classical Liberalism – another paradox. LI rests on the premise that human beings are responsive and therefore, responsible beings. LI countries find it easy and "natural" to comply with mask-wearing. However, this compliance should not be read in a merely passive manner as in the context of today's geopolitics, such compliance may also be understood as an act of Decoloniality.

Table 8.5: Differences between High Individualism and Low Individualism in respect of mask-wearing

CHAPTER 9

CONCLUSION: INTERCONNECTEDNESS AND WHOLISM

This book is an attempt to explore the interconnected complexities between the various relevant variables in the generation of any disease/illness in an individual as well as in society. It does this by focussing on one specific disease/illness, namely, SARS-CoV-2/COVID-19 whose "patient zero" may never be found and identified. However, The World Health Organisation/WHO confirmed that the Wuhan Municipal Health Commission, China, reported a cluster of cases of pneumonia in Wuhan, Hubei Province which upon further investigation was identified as having been caused by a novel coronavirus (now called the SARS-CoV-2) which has since evolved with its various variants. These cases first occurred in early December 2019 and by January of 2020, the disease/illness had moved to other cities which prompted the Chinese government to introduce a lockdown in Wuhan on 23 January 2020. The government's decision was prompted by at least three significant pieces of scientific information, namely, the pathogen causing the new disease/illness was identified as a new coronavirus by 7 January 2020, success by scientists in sequencing the virus's genome c 11 January 2020 and the announcement by the chief pulmonologist, Zhong Nanshan on 19 January 2020 that human-to-human transmission was involved.[1] The lockdown was accompanied by other measures such as testing, tracing and tracking as well as isolation of the infected, physical and/or social distancing, including mask-wearing. All such measures together enabled China officially to end the lockdown on 8 April 2020.

The Director General of the WHO was concerned enough to visit China between 16-24 February 2020 to learn first-hand about the situation there.[2] On 30 January 2020, the WHO had declared a PHEIC (Public Health

---

[1] See "Progress report on the coronavirus pandemic". *Nature*, 2020 (19 August).

[2] The visit resulted in the Report of the WHO-China Joint Mission on Coronavirus Disease 2019 (COVID-19) published on 28 February 2020. Accessed January 31, 2022. https://www.who.int/publications/i/item/report-of-the-who-china-joint-mission-on-coronavirus-disease-2019-(covid-19) .

Emergency of International Concern). However, on 11 March 2020, Dr Tedros Adhanom Ghebreyesus used the more familiar term "pandemic" to describe the phenomenon instead of the technical term "PHEIC". [3] This reality even punctured the bubble which the then President of the USA, Donald Trump had built around himself; on 17 March 2020 as he was forced to admit a pandemic was in existence in spite of an earlier denial or downplaying its seriousness when the first case of COVID-19 was reported in his country on 21 January 2020. The WHO on 26 February 2020 announced that daily new cases outside exceeded those inside China, with 2,790 cases across 37 countries and 44 deaths.

Italy, Spain, France and Germany announced their respective lockdowns on 9, 14, 17, 22 March 2020. When China officially ended the lockdown on 8 April 2020, the disease was reaching its peak in the USA. The *British Medical Journal* on 11 February 2021 published its estimate of infection and fatality in Wuhan-China: 3870 deaths (out of a total of 4600 in China) with 50,000 cases of infection in Wuhan out of c 80,000 in China.

On 14 April 2020, the US President, Donald Trump, announced that his country would stop funding the WHO on the grounds that it propagated China's misinformation about the virus which resulted in so many deaths. On 2 April 2020, Worldometer (Total cases/1 million population) listed the USA 94,026 as leading the table, followed by Sweden 80,145, Belgium 76,364, the Netherlands 75,026, Spain 70,376, France 71,810, UK 63,880, Brazil 60,099, Italy 60,088, Germany 33,056. The table then shows that the rate of infection declined dramatically in other (in the main, non-Western) countries as follows: Japan 3,784, South Korea 2,031, Hong Kong 1,525, Australia 1,149, New Zealand 500, Thailand 414, Cambodia 151, China 63, Taiwan 44, Vietnam 27. The figures for Deaths/1 million population were equally spectacular: Belgium 1,982, UK 1,861, Italy 1,821, USA 1,705, Spain 1,615, Brazil 1,523, France 1,468, Sweden 1,330, the Netherlands 966, Germany 920, Japan 73, Australia 35, South Korea 34, Hong Kong 27, New Zealand 5, China 3, Thailand 1, Cambodia 0.9, Taiwan 0.4, Vietnam 0.4. Worldometer on 29 January 2023 still shows more or less the same ranking as it did nearly three years ago: The USA 311,177 still leads with Total Cases/1 million population and 3,384 Deaths/1 million population; figures for China stand respectively at 347 and 4.

This book sets out, in the main to challenge the relationship standardly perceived between the two main domains of biomedicine, namely, Clinical Medicine on the one hand and Epidemiology on the other – the former is said to be superior and the latter somewhat substandard and inferior. This

[3] On the use of these terms "PHEIC" and "pandemic", see earlier Chapters 4 and 8.

"Cinderella" assessment of Epidemiology appears to imply an excessive deference to the achievements of giants such as Pasteur (1822-1895) and Koch (1843-1910) and their pioneering work in the germ theory of disease primarily in the nineteenth century which is considered as having introduced a paradigm shift in Medical Thinking from the humoral theory (as well as the miasma theory) of disease-causation. This is the so-called Monogenic Conception of Disease which is said to usher in the Age of Modern Medicine.[4] This book calls this the Classical Version of the Monogenic Conception of Disease. Unfortunately, for some seven decades since its appearance, it had been elevated to the status of a dogma – see Stewart 1968.

In order to challenge the Clinical Medicine-Epidemiology divide as standardly understood, one then needs to subject the Monogenic Conception of Disease (held as dogma) to critical scrutiny to see how well it might survive or how badly it might fail the test. Chapters 2, 3 and 4, therefore, set out to carry out this task, asking the following **W** questions:

1. **W**hat could be said to be the cause of the illness, called COVID-19?
2. **W**ho is likely to be infected?
3. **W**here is infection likely to take place?
4. **W**hen is infection likely to occur?

In other words, one is critically examining the Monogenic Conception of Disease held as dogma from the vantage point of its model of causation. The model underpinning it turns out to be the unidirectional, monofactorial causation/UMC, with the causal arrow leading only from Cause to Effect. UMC fails to do justice to Medical Thinking in general including Clinical Medicine in two ways: (a) by disregarding that in reality these questions are interconnected and that their interconnectedness (IC) may be summed up as the 4**W**s+IC formula.

This, then, clears the way to argue for a bidirectional, multifactorial model of causation/BMC with complicated feedback mechanisms between them – the causal arrow is minimally reciprocal, leading to a more complex network of causal connectivity. Moreover, as Mackie, 1974/1980 argued, the cause refers to a set of relevant factors related to one another in a certain way which he called "inus conditions".

---

[4] This theory took several decades (short of a full century) to have any practical impact. Alexander Fleming's chance discovery of antibiotics in 1928 was only turned into a "magic bullet" when Howard Florey and Ernst Chain managed to mass manufacture them during WWII. As a result, the Nobel Prize in Physiology and Medicine was bestowed in 1945 on Fleming, Florey and Chain.

At the risk of being repetitive and boring, it is relevant to remind readers that an adequate account of causation must consider the distinction between necessary and sufficient conditions and must refer explicitly or imply both – an account which talks only about a necessary condition, say in the context of the COVID-19 epidemic/pandemic by singling out SARS-CoV-2 as "the cause" would be highly misleading. As Stewart 1968 points out, this could happen when the Monogenic Conception of Disease/the germ theory of disease comes to be held as dogma. Held non-dogmatically, the germ theory can imply other variables which together with the germ or pathogenic factor in question can bring about the disease, constituting the necessary as well as sufficient conditions for its occurrence. These other variables can, in Stewart's words, include "susceptibility, generic constitution, behaviour, and socioeconomic determinants." (*The Lancet*, May 18, 1968, 1077). They cover variables which could be said to belong to what may be called the internal as well as the external environment of the individual who becomes infected – see, for example, Figure 3.2.

To reinforce the critique against such a conception of disease (held as dogma), this book explores Collingwood's Sense II of cause, deploying the criterion of controllability or prevention of the disease/illness in question. This demonstrates that how one picks a variable from the set of "inus conditions" cuts across the Clinical Medicine-Epidemiological divide. Sometimes, it uses a pharmaceutical strategy (falling into the domain of Clinical Medicine) but at other times and in other contexts, it uses a non-pharmaceutical or Epidemiological measure, such as lockdown, social or physical distancing, mask-wearing and so forth. In yet other contexts, to curb or control the disease/illness, the medical profession and society might resort to vaccines and vaccination if these are readily and speedily accessible and available. And yet, when the concept of vaccines is subjected to scrutiny, it turns out that it falls into both domains of biomedicine, that is, Clinical Medicine and Epidemiology. Vaccines are Janus-faced – they are manufactured in laboratories under the aegis of Clinical Medicine but are tested in the population at large under the aegis of Epidemiology. The efficacy or efficiency of a vaccine against a particular disease/illness such as COVID-19 is determined by the procedures of testing in Clinical Medicine as well as in Epidemiology.

If the above claims are plausible and cogently argued, then this book may be permitted to conclude that Medical Thinking is best presented as Ecosystem Thinking, a form of Systems Thinking, in terms of Ecosystem-nesting. Clinical Medicine ultimately works at the level of the cell in the human body. This way of looking at the nature of disease/illness means that it should not be grasped through Reductionist lenses; instead, Ecosystem

Thinking through Ecosystem-nesting (as explored in Chapter 7) embodying Wholism is the recommended correct approach. In other words, to summarise things very simplistically, one cannot fully understand how a drug can work to bring about a change or changes in cell functioning without grasping that a cell works not in isolation but in relationship with other cells. As the body of a human being is made up not only of cells, but also of tissues and organs (which themselves are constituted of cells) and that all these function in certain ways to keep the human being alive and well under normal circumstances until a pathogen subverts the functioning system. In the end, how well individual humans survive, thrive or fail to thrive depends on the complicated relationships embedded within the "ecosystems" nesting one within the other which this book has invoked, using Ecosystem-nesting in terms of concentric circles as an analytical tool.

Medicine in its two major domains of Clinical Medicine and Epidemiology embodies values, as it is an enterprise which presupposes that (other things being equal) a life of suffering pain which disease/illness often brings is something human beings would rather live without. Hence, Medical Thinking is targeted at decreasing the level of disease-generation in society. As already emphasised, while Clinical Medicine uses pharmaceutical strategies to achieve this value, Epidemiology uses non-pharmaceutical strategies to attain the same goal. As Epidemiological Thinking is less fully grasped given the "Cinderella status" it is perceived to occupy, Chapter 8 sets out to fill this gap in societal perception of this domain of biomedicine.

Chapter 8 focuses on mask-wearing to bring out the value-ladenness of Medicine – these values cover what may be called ethical, cultural, political and indeed even geopolitical values. Value differences in different philosophical-cultural traditions would therefore engage with mask-wearing (as well as lockdown) in very different ways and would account, in general, for how they handle an epidemic/pandemic such as COVID-19 in the way that they do. For instance, the US may be said to stand at one end of the Individualism spectrum and China at the opposite end – the former occupies a position which may be called the High Individualism end and the latter the Low Individualism end. As a result, some Americans are prone to regard wearing face-masks as an assault on their individual right to freedom and autonomy as self-interested persons, while the majority of Chinese people (as well as well as people of countries in the East Pacific with whom they share a common Confucian outlook) tend to regard it and other measures including lockdowns as an expression of solidarity with fellow human beings, to create a harmonious society in which the good of others is promoted even if it costs the self some inconvenience and discomfort, and even severe economic sacrifice in some cases through losing one's livelihood and loss of productivity in countries which resort to lockdowns.

It is also plausible for Low Individualism to claim that promoting solidarity and harmony is a win-win situation which not only benefits the other but also the self in the context of controlling a pandemic such as COVID-19. The logic of R (the transmission rate) dictates that the smaller the number of infected cases in the population, the lower the chance of the self being exposed to infection and being infected by such exposure. The pair of polar contrasts – self and other – is not understood dualistically (with the self being privileged over the other or with the other privileged over the self). Instead, it is understood dyadically, just as in the iconic *Yinyang* pairing where neither *yin* nor *yang* is regarded as inferior or superior. *Yin* and *yang* are different but are equal, entering into a harmonious relationship with each other to form a Whole.[5]

In other words, to understand the nature of a disease/illness, whether in more normal circumstances or in an epidemic/pandemic, Medical Thinking to do justice to its two major domains, that is, Clinical Medicine and Epidemiology, needs to invoke a Wholist philosophical-causal framework, such as that embodied in Ecosystem Thinking in terms of Ecosystem-nesting as advocated by this book.

It is also appropriate to remind the reader that in an epidemic or pandemic, the well-being of a country is not only linked with geopolitical values, but also with economic values of any one country or nation-state. Every country has to juggle with two balls to keep them up in the air at the same time, so to speak. Good governance is measured by ensuring that the nation's well-being is secured in health (relatively free from preventable sickness and death) and in economic terms (relatively prosperous). In an epidemic or pandemic, in the relatively short term, security in health may be purchased at the expense of economic flourishing – it is obvious that pursuing a zero-COVID-19 policy would save lives and suffering but would adversely affect the economic activities of the nation. There, then, comes a point in time, during an epidemic or pandemic, when health regulations may have to be relaxed in order to promote the goal of economic well-being.[6] According to an American saying: there is no such thing as a free lunch. Everything comes at a price; every policy has pluses as well as minuses. Every country/government has to make up its own mind within its own

[5] For a brief account of Wholism, see the section which follows but for a detailed exploration of the concept and related issues, see Lee, 2017.

[6] For some assessments of how China's abandonment of its zero-COVID-19 policy in economic terms has fared (up to February 2023), see Brazier and Jiang 2023; *Japan Times* (2023); *The New York Times* 2023.

moral/social/cultural framework about the balance it ought to target between these two competing, at times conflicting values. The outcomes of such targeting are different, some having done better than others.

Exploring the Values Embedded in the Concept of Wholism on the Part of Low Individualism

One ought to end with a brief section spelling out the interconnectedness of all the themes raised in the main chapters of the book (namely, Chapters 2 – 8) via the concept of Wholism. These various themes include the following:

(a) A critique of the Monogenic Conception of Disease held simplistically as dogma, explored primarily in Chapters 2, 3 and 4.
(b) Challenging the "Cinderella" status of Epidemiology and the elevation of Clinical Medicine under biomedicine, by arguing that Medical Thinking which cuts across these two domains of biomedicine is, upon critical analysis, Epidemiological Thinking – a theme which runs through all the chapters of the book.
(c) That Medical Thinking, that is, Epidemiological Thinking is Wholist in orientation, a theme explored in detail in Chapter 7, via the notion of Ecosystem-nesting.

Chapter 8 (see Table 8.5) has distinguished between High Individualism at one end of the spectrum and Low Individualism at the other. It also postulates that while the USA may be seen as an exemplification of High Individualism, China may be seen as an exemplification of Low Individualism. This section would now like to develop Low Individualism further by seeing it as an instantiation of the concept of Wholism. Wholism can be understood as a metaphysical concept which nonetheless embodies certain norms and values. Some of its characteristics have already been alluded to in Chapters 1 and 7. Put simplistically, it may be set out as follows, bearing in mind the distinction made in Chapter 1 between "whole/ wholism", "Whole/Wholism":

(a) A whole has constituent parts; so does a Whole.
(b) What distinguishes a whole from a Whole, is the respective relations between them and their constituent parts.
(c) A whole is said to be no more than the sum of its constituent parts; on the other hand, a Whole is more than or is different from the sum of its constituent parts.

Here are some mundane and familiar examples of wholes and Wholes. You are trying to make a drink for which you need some sugar, some mint and some hot water, according to your recipe. When you've collected these three items on your kitchen table, you have a whole; should you change your mind, you can dismantle this whole quite easily by putting each of its constituent items to other different uses. The properties of these ingredients remain the same. However, once you have put the mint, the sugar in a jug and added hot water to them, you have produced a Whole which you cannot dismantle or deconstruct, restoring each constituent ingredient to its original properties. The drink, the Whole has what philosophers call emergent properties[7] which cannot be reduced to the sum of the properties of the ingredients as separate entities. The taste of such a drink is different from that of the sugar, the mint or the hot water when each is tasted separately. In the same way a cake is a Whole as its properties are emergent properties which are different from the sum of the properties of its individual raw ingredients such as the sugar, the eggs, the flour. If you were to eat some sugar, an egg and some flour, you have not eaten a cake – a cake has its own texture and taste as well as appearance (in terms of its shape and size) which cannot be reduced to those of its separate ingredients, although they have each contributed to the final outcome, the cake.

One could use the distinction between a mixture and a compound in chemistry to say that a compound is a Whole, whereas a mixture is a whole. Take a molecule of water, which is a compound, made up of two atoms of hydrogen and one atom of oxygen (H_2O). Water, unlike its constituent atoms, is wet, can quench thirst, put out a fire and so forth which its constituent parts each on its own does not possess. Hence, we can say that a compound is really a Whole, as this compound has properties which are different from or more than the sum of its constituent parts, its atoms. On the other hand, a solution of salt water is a mixture as one can recover the two constituents from the solution, and there is no fixed ratio with its properties depending solely on the properties of its constituent parts – it is therefore according to the terminology of this book, a whole, not a Whole.

A handful of stones (identical in shape, size and colour) and a handful of soil can also usefully serve to illustrate the difference between the two terms, "wholism" and "Wholism" and the concepts standing behind them. If one has 5 such stones and one were to arrange them in a certain pattern; the pattern constitutes a whole. One can dismantle it and construct another pattern, another whole and nothing would be lost. On the other hand, a handful of soil, which constitutes a Whole, has a past, a present and a future

[7] For one philosophically detailed account, see O'Connor 2021 (Winter).

in ecological terms. Imagine yourself walking through an ancient forest; you bend down and scoop up from the forest floor a handful of soil. That handful of soil is the product of long evolutionary processes of change and development between its various constituent parts, such as bacteria and other micro-organisms which may live in the soil (its biota), the tiny particles of abiotic Nature which have taken centuries if not millennia to weather down from the original rocks (which may even have been hard granite) through the action of heat, cold, wind, the roots of other plants in its vicinity, animals big and small trampling over it, and so forth. You cannot, however, dismantle or deconstruct the soil into its original separate constituent parts without destroying the Whole; nor can you construct another Whole from such separate constituent parts, even if you can correctly identify them and lay your hands on them. And even if you could assemble them together and wait several centuries if not millennia to see if a new Whole would appear, that Whole of this imagined future might not bear too much resemblance to the Whole right now in the palm of your hands – the micro-organisms might not be identical, the climate might have altered with longer, hotter summers or longer, colder winters, factors which are relevant to the emergence of the soil with its characteristics and properties.

Another familiar example of a Whole is a bee colony such as that of the honeybee. Such a colony typically consists of three types of bees: the drones, the queen and the most numerous members of the colony, the workers. The drones which are males perform the one important function of fertilising the queen to maintain reproduction. The queen performs two functions: laying eggs (and hence plays an indispensable role in reproduction) as well as producing pheromones to provide a specific social glue for the colony, shaping the behaviour of the other bees. The largest constituent of the colony is the worker bee, a sexually under-developed female whose roles are numerous, including the cleaning of the nest/hive (maintaining proper hygiene standards, safeguarding the health of the entire colony), the collection of pollen from the surrounding flowering plants as well as performing the waggle dance to inform fellow workers where exactly the best pollen may be found (putting food on the table for the colony, so to speak), the security of the colony by guarding its entrance against invaders which can damage the colony.

Society for High Individualism is a whole which contains no more than the sum of the individuals found within its boundaries. Each individual is a self-contained social atom and is typically motivated to advance its own perceived interests. Society for Low Individualism is a Whole whose constituents embrace, as we have seen, duties and obligations to Others, seeing themselves bound to societal norms, such as: "don't do anything which can put your community/society/country to shame or at risk", "advance the common good even if it may mean inconvenience to the self or even sacrificing oneself for the safety/security of the community/society/country. For Low Individualists or Wholists, advancing common safety, security or prosperity is a shared value. It is not sufficient that oneself should survive, thrive or flourish but fellow members of the tribe, community, society, country should do so. In the words of Ingold, Low Individualists are "responsive beings".

Mask-wearing asks Low Individualists to sacrifice their own inconvenience for the good of others. Lockdowns demand even a greater degree of self-sacrifice as Low Individualists are asked to restrict their freedom of movement and activity, including in many instances their livelihood, for the sake of protecting the community at large from being exposed to the virus and to the damage to health that such exposure could cause.

However, the nature of Epidemiological Thinking and its strategies also ensure a win-win situation – as lockdowns and mask-wearing reduce the transmission of the virus in the community/country, this means that the opportunities of exposure and of infection would be much less. All is not self-sacrifice, as the self can benefit from the collective good of controlling/decreasing the transmission rate of the virus in the community/country. Interconnectedness is all.

REFERENCES AND SELECT BIBLIOGRAPHY

Adam, David. 2023 (1 February). "When will COVID stop being a global emergency?" *Nature Briefing*. Accessed February 3, 2023, https://www.nature.com/articles/d41586-023-00294-9?utm_source= Nature+ Brief ing&utm _campaign

"America's CDC abruptly changes its guidance on face-masks. 2021 (17 May)", *The Economist*. Accessed May 17, 2021, https://www.economist.com/graphic-detail/2021/05/17/americas-cdc-abruptly-changes-its-guidance-on-face-masks

Amnesty International Report. 2020 (4 October). *UK: Older people in care homes abandoned to die amid government failures during COVID-19 pandemic*. Accessed July 10, 2022, https://www.amnesty. org/ en/ latest/press-release/2020/ 10/ uk-older-people-in-care-homes-abandon ed-to-die-amid-government-failures-during-covid-19-pandemic/

Angell, Marcia. 2004, *The Truth About the Drug Companies: How They Deceive Us and What To Do About It*, New York: Random House

Auwaerter, Paul Gisbert, and Casadevall, Arturo. 2022 (15 June), "Treatment for Covid", *John Hopkins Medicine*. Accessed September 22, 2022, https://www.hopkinsmedicine.org/health/conditions-and-diseases/coronavirus/ coronavirus-treatment-whats-in-development

Baggini, Julian. 2018. *How the World Thinks: A Global History of Philosophy*, London: Granta Books

Bai, Y., Yao, L., Wei, T., Tian, F., Chen, L., and Wang, M. 2020 (14 April) "Presumed Asymptomatic Carrier Transmission of COVID-19". *Journal of the American Medical Association* 323(14):1406-1407. Accessed May 12, 2023, https://jamanetwork.com/searchresults?q = Presum-ed%20Asymptomatic%20Carrier%20Transmission%20of% 20COVID-19.&allSites=1&SearchSourceType=1&exPrm_qqq= {DE FAULT_ BOOST_ FUNCTION}% 22 Presumed% 20 Asymptoma tic%20Carrier%20Transmission%20of%20COVID-19

Bardi, Jason Socrates. 2009 (14 June) "The Gross Science of a Cough and a Sneeze" *Live Science*. Accessed August 8, 2021, https://www.livescience.com/3686-gross-science-cough-sneeze.html

BBC News. 2020 (12 July). "Coronavirus: Donald Trump wears face mask for the first time". Accessed August 12, 2021, https:// www. bbc.co.uk/news/world-us-canada-53378439

BBC Two. Horizon. 2010 (20 January), "Pill Poppers". Accessed August 15, 2022, https://www.bbc.co.uk/ programmes/b00q9jfs

Bhopal, Raj S. 2002/2008. *Concepts of Epidemiology: An Integrated Introduction to the Ideas, Theories, Principles and Methods of Epidemiology*, Oxford: Oxford University Press

Biswas, Soutik. 2022 (5 May). "Why India's real Covid toll may never be known", BBC. Accessed September 26, 2022, https://www.bbc.co.uk/ news/world-asia-india-6098 13 18

Bloom, Jesse D.2023 (25 April). "Association between SARS-CoV-2 and metagenomic content of samples from the Huanan Seafood Market". *bioRxiv*. Accessed May 11, 2023, https://www.biorxiv.org/content/ 10.1101/2023.04.25.538336v1.full.pdf

Booth, Robert. 2023 (28 February). "UK Covid inquiry urged to consider structural racism in every part of investigation. Almost all minority ethnic groups were more likely to die from virus than white British people", *The Guardian*. Accessed February 28, 2023, https://www. the guardian.com/uk-news/2023/feb/28/uk-covid-inquiry-urged-to-consi der-structural-racism-in-every-part-of-investigation

Brazier, Alex and Jiang, Serena. 2023 (February 21). "China reopening: growth spurt, policy pivot and long-term challenges", Blackrock Investment Institute. Accessed May 2, 2023, https://www.blackrock. com/corporate/insights/blackrock-investment-institute/economic-insights/2023/02/china-reopening-growth-spurt

Broadbent, Alex. 2013. *Philosophy of Epidemiology*, Basingstoke: Palgrave Macmillan

Broadbent, Lindsay. 2023 (19 July). "COVID: a gene mutation could help explain why some people don't get symptoms – new research", *The Conversation*. Accessed July 20, 2023, COVID: a gene mutation could help explain why some people don't get symptoms – new research (theconversation.com)

Brothers, Will. 2020 (3 December). "A Timeline of COVID-19 Vaccine Development", *BioSpace*. Accessed February 15, 2022, https://www. biospace.com/article/a-timeline-of-covid-19-vacc ine-development/

Buckley, Chris, and Chang, Chien Amy. 2023 (31 January). "As China's Covid Tsunami Recedes, Relief, Grief and Anxiety Follow", *The New York Times*. Accessed February 1, 2023, https://www.nytimes.com/ 2023/01/31/ world/asia/china-covid-infections-decrease.html

Carter, K. Codell. 2003. *The Rise of Causal Concepts in Disease: Case Histories*, Aldershot: Ashgate Publishing Limited

CDC, USA. 2021 (7 May). "Scientific brief: Community use of cloth masks to control the spread of SARS-CoV-2", The National Center for

Immunization and Respiratory Diseases (US), Division of Viral Diseases. Accessed July 16, 2022, https://stacks.cdc.gov/view/cdc/105951

Chang, Phoebe. 2023 (29 January). "China reports sharp drop in Covid deaths during Lunar New Year holiday", *South China Morning Post*. Accessed February 5, 2023, https://www.scmp.com/news/china/ science/article/3208357/china-reports-sharp-drop-covid-deaths-during-lunar-new-year-holiday

Chen, Simiao, Zhang Zongjiu, Yang Juntao, Wang Jian, Zhai Xiaohui, Till Bärnighausen, Till and Chen Wang. 2020 (2 April). "Fangcang shelter hospitals: a novel concept for responding to public health emergencies", *The Lancet*. Accessed May 23, 2021, https://www.Fangcang shelter hospitals: a novel concept for responding to public health emergencies - The Lancet

—. *The Covid-19 Commission*, *The Lancet* 10 October 2020, Vol 396: 1102-1124

Chen, Tina. 2021 (23 March). "Fomites and the COVID-19 pandemic: An evidence review on its role in viral transmission", National Collaborating Centre for Environmental Health/ *Centre de collaboration nationale en santé environmentale*. Accessed September 19, 2021, http://Fomites and the COVID-19 pandemic: An evidence review on its role in viral transmission | National Collaborating Centre for Environmental Health | NCCEH - CCSNE

Cheng, Kar Keung, Lam Tai Hing, and Leung Chi Chiu. 2020 (14 April). "Wearing face masks in the community during the COVID-19 pandemic: altruism and solidarity", *The Lancet*. Accessed August 7, 2021, http://Wearing face masks in the community during the COVID-19 pandemic: altruism and solidarity - The Lancet

"China must share data on COVID-19's origins 'immediately' WHO scientist demands", 2023 (6 April). WHO. Accessed April 7, 2023, https://www.livescience.com/china-must-share-data-on-covid-19s-origins-immediately-who-scientist-demands

Chow, Denise. 2021 (1 September). "Largest study of masks yet details their importance in fighting Covid-19", NBCNEWS, (Preprint study posted online by Innovations for Poverty Action). Accessed January 2, 2022, http://Largest study of masks yet details their importance in fighting Covid-19 (nbcnews.com)

CNN. 2021 (8 January). "Taiwan's COVID-19 Enforcement Success Includes Quarantine Hotels, Musical Trash Trucks". Accessed August 8, 2021, https://edition.cnn.com/2020/07/27/asia/hong-kong-masks-coronavirus-restrictions-intl-hnk/ index

Cochrane, A. L. 1972 (1999), *Effectiveness and Efficiency: Random reflections on Health Services.* 1st ed. London: Nuffield Trust, Cambridge: The Royal Society of Medicine Press Limited

Cohen, J. 2017. *Infectious Diseases* (Fourth Edition), Volume 1, *The Evolution of Koch's Postulates. Section 1*: Introduction to Infectious Diseases. Accessed April 5, 2023, https://reader.elsevier.com/reader/sd/pii/B9780702062858000010? token=75BBA8D30D3AAA0931 D9 4E 6E45663F18E3B6EC5176AC3C21150917453E417866FFC5744C 687BEC0291DB03DE473B50A0&originRegion=eu-west-1&origin Creation=20230405211257

Collingwood, R. G. 1938. "The So Called Idea of Causation", *Proceedings of the Aristotelian Society*, Volume 85. 1938, 85-112

"Consensus Development Conference Statement: Helicobacter Pylori in Peptic Ulcer Disease", National Institutes of Health 1994 (7-9 February). Accessed April 5, 2022, https://consensus.nih.gov/1994/1994HelicobacterPyloriUlcer 094html.htm

"COVID-19 Therapeutics. n.d." AAFP / The American Academy of Family Physicians Foundation. Accessed February 6, 2023, https://www.aafp.org/about/policies/all/prescription-covid19.html

"COVID-origins data from Wuhan market published: what scientists think" 2023 (5 April). *Nature News*. Accessed April 6, 2023, https://www.nature.com/articles/d41586-023-00998-y

"COVID-19 Vaccines". 2023 (17 February). WHO. Accessed February 26, 2023, https://www.who.int/westernpacific/emergencies/covid-19/covid-19-vaccines

Cramer, Maria and Sheikh, Knvul. 2020 (February 29), updated 2021 (September 12), "Surgeon General Urges the Public to Stop Buying Face Masks". *The New York Times*. Accessed October 15, 2022, https:// www.nytimes.com/2020/02/29/health/coronavirus-n95-face-masks.html

Criado Perez, C. 2019. *Invisible Women: Data Bias in a World Designed for Men*, London: Chatto and Windus

Daniels, Marc, and Bradford Hill, A. 1952. "Chemotherapy of Pulmonary Tuberculosis in Young Adults: An Analysis of the Combined Results of Three Medical Research Council Trials", *The British Medical Journal*, 1 May (4769): 1162-1168. Accessed October 24, 2022, https://www.bmj.com/content/1/4769/1162

De, Kai, Goldstein, Guy-Philippe, Morgunov, Alexey, Nangalia, Vishal, and Rotkirch, Anna. 2020 (22 April), "Universal Masking is Urgent in the COVID-19 Pandemic: SEIR and Agent Based Models, Empirical

Validation, Policy Recommendations", (arXiv2004.13553v1 [physics.soc-ph]. Accessed April 14, 2023, https://arxiv.org/abs/2004.13553

—. 2020 (24 April). "Universal Masking to Restart Society and Save Lives: COVID-19 Data, Simulations, Policy Recommendations". Accessed August 18, 2021, http://dek.ai/masks4all/ universal masking. pdf.

Dey, Sushmi. 2020 (7 April). "63% of Covid-19 deaths in India among 60-plus". *The Times of India*. Accessed July 10, 2022, https://www. Coronavirus deaths in India: 63% of Covid-19 deaths in India among 60-plus | India News - Times of India (indiatimes.com)

"Did the COVID-19 lockdowns work? Here's what we know two years on" 2022 (March 23), *The Conversation*. Accessed April 13, 2023, https:// theconversation. com/did-the-covid-lockdowns-work-heres-what-we-know-two-years-on-1766 23

Diez Roux, Ana. 2011. "Complex Systems Thinking and Current Impasses in Health Disparities Research", *American Journal of Public Health*, 101(9): 1627-1634

Eds. Gina S. Lovasi, Ana V. Diez Roux and Jennifer Kolker. 2021, "Conceptual Models and Frameworks for Understanding the Links Between Urban Environments and Health", *Urban Public Health*. Oxford: Oxford University Press

Dusenbery, Maya. 2017. *Doing Harm: The Truth About How Bad Medicine and Lazy Science Leave Women Dismissed, Misdiagnosed, and Sick,* New York: HarperOne

Ellis-Petersen, Hannah 2023 (April 13). *The Guardian*. Accessed April 16, 2023. See also: "India increases Covid booster jab production after surge in cases", 2023 (12 April). Accessed April 16, 2023, https://www.theguardian.com/world/2023/apr/12/india-increases-covid-booster-jab-production-after-surge-in-cases

"Epidemic, Endemic, Pandemic: What are the Differences?" 2021 (February 19), Columbia University Irving Medical Center. Accessed August 16, 2022, https://www.public health.columbia.edu/public-health -now/news/epidemic-endemic-pandemic-what-are-differences

Erath, Byron D., and Ferro, Andrea R. 2022 (12 September). "Infectious disease transmission from bioaerosols", *Journal of Exposure Science & Environmental Epidemiology*, 32, 545-646

Evans, Alfred S. 1976. (May). "Causation and Disease: The Henle-Koch Postulated Revisited", *Yale J. Biol. Med.* 49(2): 175-195. Accessed May 14, 2021, https://www.ncbi.nlm.nih.gov/pmc/articles/PMC2595276/

—. 1993. *Causation and Disease: A Chronological Journey,* New York: Plenum

Evans, David. 2002. "Hierarchy of evidence: a framework for ranking evidence evaluating healthcare interventions", *Journal of Clinical Nursing.* Accessed September 18, 2021, https:/ /online library. wiley. com/doi/10.1046/j.1365-2702. 2003. 006 6 2.x

Faber, Knud Helge. 1978. *Nosography: The Evolution of Modern Internal Clinical Medicine*, New York: AMS Press

Falush, Daniel. 2020 (20 April). "Isolate, isolate, isolate: China's approach to Covid-19 quarantine could be the most effective", *The Telegraph*. Accessed July 9, 2022, https://Isolate, isolate, isolate: China's approach to Covid-19 quarantine could be the most effective (telegraph.co.uk)

Farrar, Jeremy with Ahuja, Anjana. 2021. *Spike: The Virus vs the People. The Inside Story*, London: Profile Books Ltd

Fedak, Kristen M., Bernal, Autumn, Capshaw, Zachary A., and Gross, Sherilyn. 2015 (30 September), "Applying the Bradford Hill criteria in the 21st century: how data integration has changed causal inference in molecular epidemiology", *Emerging Themes in Epidemiology*, Doi: 10.1186/s12982-015-0037-4. Accessed August 23, 2021, https:// pubmed. ncbi.nlm. nih. gov/ 26425136/

Fink, Jenni. 2020 (27 October). "Fact Check: Is a Mask Mandate Unconstitutional?" *Newsweek*. Accessed February 3, 2022, https://www. newsweek.com/fact-check-mask-mandate-unconstitutional-1542465

Finn, John E. 2020 (23 July). "No, mask mandates are not unconstitutional. Commentary", *Chicago Tribune*. Accessed August 12, 2021, https:// www.chicagotribune.com/opinion/commentary/ct-opinion-coronavirus -mask-mandates-constitution al-2020 0723-53dpqip7lff55o5fp 444mq l6cm-story.html

Full Fact. 2021 (14 July). "New study estimates mask wearing could cut R number by 25% not 0.25". Accessed August 8, 2021, https:// full fact.org/online/andy-burnham-mayor-manchester-masks-misquote/

Garner, Sarah, and Thomas, Rachel. 2010 (3 March). "Evaluating a Medical Treatment–how do you know it works", *Plus*. Accessed August 23, 2021, https://plus.maths.org/content/evaluating-medical-treatment-how-do-you-know-it-works

Glanz, James, Hvistendahl, Mara, and Chang, Agnes. 2023 (15 February) "Two months after China ended "zero Covid," rough estimates suggest that between 1 and 1.5 million people died – far more than the official count", *The New York Times.* Accessed February 16, 2023, https://www. nytimes.com/interactive/2023/02/15/world/asia/china-covid-death-estimates.html?campaign_id=51&emc=edit_mbe_20230216& instance_id=85500&nl=morning-briefing%3A-europe-edition &regi _ id=161238284&segment_id=125444&te=1&user_id=373a935f3ce481 2abad 6007c 0111 ff79

Greenberg, Jon, and Sherman, Amy. 2021 (19 January). "Timeline: How Donald Trump responded to the coronavirus pandemic", *Politifact.* Accessed August 12, 2021, https://www. politifact.com/article/2020/ mar/20/how-donald-trump-responded-coronavirus-pandemic/

Greenhaigh, Trish. 2021 (13 July). "COVID: seven reasons mask wearing in the west was unnecessarily delayed", *The Conversation.* Accessed August 8, 2021, https://theconversation.com/covid-seven-reasons-mask-wearing-in-the-west-was-unnecessarily-delayed-164308?utm_ medium

Gregory, Andrew. 2022 (15 May). "Taboo stops south Asian people in UK seeking help for dementia, says charity", *The Guardian.* Accessed August 5, 2022, https://www.theguardian.com/ society/2022/ may/ 15/ taboo-stops-south-asian-people-in-uk-seeking-help-for-dementia-says-charity

Griffiths, James. 2020 (13 October). "South Korea mandates mask-wearing to fight Covid-19 as face coverings remain controversial in the US", CNN. Accessed August 8, 2021, https://edition.cnn.com/2020/10/13/ asia/ south-korea-masks-coronavirus-intl-hnk/index.html

Grimley, Naomi, Cornish, Jack, and Stylianou, Nassos. 2022 (5 May) "Covid: World's true pandemic death toll nearly 15 million, says WHO", BBC News. Accessed September 11, 2022, https://www.bbc.co.uk/ news/health-61327778

Hammond, Phil. 2021, *Dr Hammond's Covid Casebook*, London: Private Eye Productions Limited

Harris, Richard. 2020 (16 December), "Oxygen-Detecting Devices Give Misleading Readings In People With Dark Skin", *NPR Health Newsletter.* Accessed May 14, 2022, https://www.npr.org/2020/12/16/ 947261192/oxygen-detecting-devices-give-misleading-readings-in-people-with-dark-skin?t=16525 50860733

Harrison, Neil, and Sachs, Jeffrey. 2022 (19 May), "A call for an independent inquiry into the origin of the SARS-CoV-2 virus", *Proceedings of the National Academy of Sciences*, Vol. 119, No.21. Accessed June 4, 2022, https://www.pnas.org/doi/ 10.1073/ pnas. 2202769119 .

Hayek, Friedrich. 1944, *The Road to Serfdom*, Chicago: University of Chicago Press

Head, Michael.2023 (10 March). "Three years on, the COVID pandemic may never end – but the public health impact is becoming more manageable". *The Conversation.* Accessed March 13, 2023, https:// theconversation.com/three-years-on-the-covid-pandemic-may-never-end-but-the-pub-lic-health-impact-is-becoming-more-manageable-198013

Healy, David. 2009, *The Creation of Psychopharmacology*, Cambridge, MA: Harvard University Press

Hejazi, Alireza. n. d. "You Must Know Guide to Systems Thinking". Accessed December 20, 2022, https://www.academia.edu/1841998/Your_Must_Know_Guide_to_Systems_Thinking

Hofstede, Geert. 1980. *Culture's Consequences: International Differences in Work-Related Values*. Beverly Hills, CA: Sage. 2nd Edition. 2001, *Culture's Consequences: Comparing Values, Behaviors, Institutions, and Organizations Across Nations*, Thousand Oaks, CA: Sage

—. "CLEARLY CULTURAL: Making Sense of Cross-Cultural Communication", n.d. Accessed August 18, 2022, https://clearlycultural.com/geert-hofstede-cultural-dimensions/individualism/

Ho, Peng Yoke. 1972. "The System of the *Book of Changes* and Chinese Science", *Japanese Studies in the History of Science* 11:38

Hogberg, David. 2020 (23 June). "'Culture war': Gallup finds Democrats and Republicans parting ways on social distancing", *The Washington Examiner*. Accessed August 11, 2021, https://www.Washingtonexaminer.com/news/culture-war-gallup-finds-democrats-and-republicans-parting-ways-on-social-distancing-and-masks

Hooper, David. 2020 (31 May). "HOW IS SARS-COV-2 TRANSMITTED?" Massachusetts General Hospital. Accessed August 20, 2021, https:// advances. massgeneral.org/research-and-innovation/ article. aspx? Id = 1284

Horsten, Leon, and Weber, Erik. 2005. "INUS Conditions". *Encyclopedia of Statistics in Behavioral Science,* October 2005. Accessed November 15, 2022, https:// www. researchgate. net/ publication /2294522 54 _ INUS_ Conditions

Horton, Richard. 2021. 2nd Edition, *The COVID-19 Catastrophe: WHAT'S GONE WRONG AND HOW TO STOP IT HAPPENING AGAIN,* Cambridge: Polity Press

"How Masks Went From Don't Wear to Must-Have". 2020 (July 2), *Wired*. Accessed October 12, 2022, https://www.wired.com/story/how-masks-went-from-dont-wear-to-must-have/

Howard, Jeremy, Huang, Austin, Li, Zhiyuan, + 15, and Rimoin, Anne W. 2021 (11 January) "An evidence review of face masks against COVID-

19". *Proceedings of the National Academy of Sciences*. Accessed September 18, 2021, https://www.pnas.org/doi/10.1073/pnas.2014 564118

Hutton, Mercedes. 2022 (18 March). "Hong Kong Covid crisis; why is the death rate so high?" *The Guardian*. Accessed July 9, 2022, https: // www.theguardian.com/world/2022/mar/18/hong-kong-covid-crisis-why-is -the-death-rate-so-high

Ing, N. 2005 (23 February), "Steroid Hormones Regulate Gene Expression Posttranscriptionally by Altering the Stabilities of Messenger RNAs", *Biology of Reproduction*, Vol. 72, Issue 6, 1290-1296,

Ingold, Tim. 2017. "On human correspondence", *Journal of the Royal Anthropological Institute,* Volume 23, Issue 1, 9-27. Accessed August 16, 2021, https://On human correspondence - Ingold - 2017 - Journal of the Royal Anthropological Institute - Wiley Online Library

Japan Times. 2023 (1 March), Chia's economy shows strong recovery as 'zero-COVID' era ends. Accessed 3 May 2023, https://www.japantimes.co.jp/news/2023/03/01/business/china-economy-post-covid -zero/

Jefferson, Tom. 2007, "Why the MRC randomized trials of whooping cough (pertussis) vaccines remain important more than half a century after they were done", *Journal of the Royal Society of Medicine*, 100(7): 343-345

Johnson, Robert, and Cureton, Adam. "Kant's moral philosophy (section 4)", *Stanford Encyclopedia of Philosophy* (Spring 2022 Edition), Edward N. Zalta (ed.). Accessed July 10, 2022, https://plato.stanford.edu/ archives/ spring2022/entries/kant-moral/

Kermack, W. O., and McKendrick, A.G. 1927, "A Contribution to the Mathematical Theory of Epidemics", *Proceedings of The Royal Society*. Accessed August 18, 2021, https://royalsocietypublishing.org/ doi/ pdf/ 10.1098/ rspa.1927.0118

Kostoe, Simon. 2020 (14 July), "Does your face mask protect you or other people?" *The Conversation*. Accessed August 8, 2021, https:// theconversation.com/does-your-face-mask-protect-you-or-other-people-142612

Kucharski, Adam. 2020, *The Rules of Contagion: Why Things Spread - and Why They Stop*, London: Profile

—. 2022 (23 October), "Fragmented outbreak data will lead to a repeat of COVID-19: to break the vicious cycle of patchy understanding and poor virus control, we need to talk about privacy", *Nature* 608, 649. Accessed November 25, 2022, https://www.nature.com/ articles/ d4 586-022-02 268-9?error=cookies_ not_supported&code= 383b0d733 fe8-485e-bd 9 d-f47e093614ae.

La Rosa, Giuseppina, Mancini, Pamela, Ferraro, Giusy Bonanno, Veneri, Carolina, Iaconelli, Marcello, Bonadonna, Lucia, Lucentini, Luca, and Suffredini, Elisabetta. 2021 (1 January), "SARS-CoV-2 has been circulating in northern Italy since December 2019: Evidence from environmental monitoring", *Science of the Total Environment* 750: 141711

Lai, Shengjie, and Tatem, Andrew J. 2023 (27 January), "What effect will lunar new year have on COVID spread in China? Our modelling shows most people have already been infected", *The Conversation*. Accessed January 30, 2023, https://theconversation.com/what-effect-will-lunar-new-year-have-on-covid-spread-in-china-our-modelling-shows-most-people-have-already-been-infected

Lee, Amber. 2023 (19 February), "China won't see new Covid wave despite arrival of highly contagious Omicron variant, medical expert says", *South China Morning Post*. Accessed February 20, 2023, https://www. scmp.com /news/ china/ science/article/3210759/china-wont-see-new-covid-wave-despite-arrival-highly-contagious-omicron-variant-medical-expert-says

Lee, Keekok. 2012, *The Philosophical Foundations of Modern Medicine*, Basingstoke: Palgrave Macmillan

— 2017, *The Philosophical Foundations of Classical Chinese Medicine: Philosophy, Methodology, Science,* Lanham: Lexington Press

— 2017a, "RCTs & EBM as Gold Standards: A Trojan Horse for Biomedicine?" *Knowing and Acting in Medicine* edited by Robyn Bluhm. Lanham: Rowen and Littlefield International

— 2019 (26 February), "Epidemiology is Ecosystem Science", *Synthese*, 198(10), 2539-2567; doi: 10.1007/s11229-019-02129-5, Accessed September 20, 2022, https://www.ncbi.nlm.nih.gov/pmc/articles/PMC7088955/

— forthcoming. "Addendum: Technology and De-humanization of Medicine' in *Handbook of the Philosophy of Medicine.* Second edition. edited by Thomas Schramme and Mary Walker. Dordrecht: Springer.

Leech, Gavin, Rogers-Smith, Charlie, Sandbrink, Jonas B., Zinkov, Robert, Rader, Benjamin, Brownstein, John S., Gal, Yarin, Bhatt, Samir, Sharma, Mrinank, Minermann, Sören, Brauner, Jan M., and Aitchison, Laurence. 2021 (18 June), "Mass mask-wearing notably reduces COVID-19 transmission", *Medical Review xiv*. Accessed September 4, 2021. Mass mask-wearing notably reduces COVID-19 transmission — University of Bristol

Lewis, Dyani. 2022 (7 September), "What scientists have learnt from COVID lockdowns: Restrictions on social contact stemmed disease spread, but weighing up the ultimate costs and benefits of lockdown measures is a challenge", *Nature* 609, 236-239. Accessed November 5, 2022, https://www.nature.com/articles/d41586-022-02823-4?utm_source=Nature+Briefing&utmcampaign=4a8f0a18ec-briefing-dy-20220907&utm_medium=email&utm_term=0_c9dfd39373-4a8f0a18ec-45880058

Livingston, Paul and Cainer, Joshua. 2022 (29 July), "UK Covid-19 inquiry launches with OTC members on legal teams", Outer Temple. Accessed September 20, 2022, https://www.outertemple.com/uk-covid-19-inquiry-launches-with-otc-members-on-legal-team/

Ma, Q., Liu, J., Liu, Q., Kang, L., Liu, R., Jing, W., Wu, Y. and Liu, Min. 2021 (14 December), "Global Percentage of Asymptomatic SARS-CoV-2 Infections Among the Tested Population and Individuals with Confirmed COVID-19 Diagnosis", *Jama* Network, Open Access. Accessed November 18, 2022, https://jamanetwork.com/ journals/ jamanetwork open/ fullarticle/2787098

MacGill, Markus. 2018 (4 December), "What is a randomized controlled trial?" *Medical News Today*. Accessed September 19, 2022, https:// www. medicalnewstoday.com/articles/280574#what-is-a-ran domized -controlled-trial

Mackie, John Leslie. 1965, "Causes and Conditions", *American Philosophical Quarterly*, 12: 245-65

—. 1974/1980, *The Cement of the Universe: A Study of Causation*, Oxford: Oxford University Press

Macleod, Christopher. 2016 (25 August), "John Stuart Mill". *The Stanford Encyclopedia of Philosophy*, Edward N. Zalta (ed.). Accessed March 12, 2022, https://plato.stanford.edu/entries/mill/

Mahbubani, Kishore. 2022. "Can Humanity Make U-turns?" *The Asian 21st Century: China and Globalization*. New York: Springer.

Maher, Brendan, and Van Noorden, Richard. 2021, "How the COVID pandemic is changing global science collaborations: The pandemic and political tensions might slow the march towards more globalised science", *Nature* 594, 316-319. Accessed September 22, 2022, http://doi.org/ 10.1038/d41586-021-01570-2

Mallapaty, Smriti. 2023 (14 February), "WHO abandons plans for crucial second phase of COVID-origins investigation", *Nature Briefing*. Accessed February 14, 2023, https://www.nature.com/ articles/d41586-023-00283-y?utm_source= Nature+ Briefing&utm_ campaign= 4cb 84 e684e-briefing-dy-20230214&utm_medium= email& utmterm=0_ c9d fd39 373-4cb 84e 68 4e-45880058

Maragakis, Lisa. 2021 (3 June), "Can wearing a face mask prevent coronavirus from spreading?" *Johns Hopkins Medicine*. Accessed August 6, 2021, https://www.hopkinsmedicine.org/health/conditions-and-diseases/corona virus/corona virus-face-masks-what-you-need-to-know

Mathew, Cynthia. 2019 (10 August), "Not All Viruses Are Bad For You. Here Are Some That Can Have a Protective Effect", *The Conversation*. Accessed: January 9, 2023, Not All Viruses Are Bad For You. Here Are Some That Can Have a Protective Effect : ScienceAlert

Mayo Clinic Staff. 2021 (4 August), "How well do face masks protect against coronavirus?" The Mayo Clinic. Accessed August 6, 2021, https://www. mayoclinic.org/diseases-conditions/coronavirus/in-depth/ coronavirus-mask/ art-20485449

McKelvey, Tara. 2020 (20 July), "Coronavirus: why are Americans so angry about masks". Accessed August 10, 2021, https://www. bbc. co. uk/news/world-us-canada-53477121

Medical Xpress. 2020 (September 7), "China shows off COVID-19 vaccines for the first time". Accessed February 15, 2022, https:// medicalxpress.com/news/2020-09-china-covid-vaccines.html

Mignolo, Walter. 2017, Part 1 (Activism and Trajectory) and Part 2 (Key Concepts), Interviews conducted by Alvina Hoffman, and editor at E-IR. Accessed February 19, 2022, https://www.e-ir.info/2017/01/17/ interview-walter-mignolopart-1-activism-and-trajectory/ ; https://www. e-ir.info/ 2017/01/21/interview-walter-mignolopart-2-key-concepts/# google _vignette

Mill, John Stuart. 1974, *A System of Logic*. Toronto and London: University of Toronto Press, Routledge and Kegan Paul. Accessed February 5, 2022, http://www.gutenberg.org/etext/27942

Mueller, Benjamin.2023 (March 16), "New Data Links Pandemic's Origins to Racoon Dogs at Wuhan Market", *The New York Times*. Accessed March 17, 2023, https://www.nytimes.com/2023/03/16/science/covid-wuhan-market-raccoon-dogs-lab-leak.html?campaign_id= 190&emc = edit_ufn_20230317&instance_id=87938&nl=from-the-times&regi_id= 161238284&segment_id=128011&te=1&user_id=373a935f3ce4812ab ad6007c0111ff79

Nakayachi, Kazuya, Ozaki, Taku, and Shibata, Yukihide. 2020 (4 August), "Why Japanese People Use Masks Against COCID-19, Even Though Masks Are Unlikely to Offer Protection From Infection?" *Frontiers in Psychology*. Accessed August 15, 2021, Frontiers | Why Do Japanese People Use Masks Against COVID-19, Even Though Masks Are Unlikely to Offer Protection From Infection? | Psychology (frontiersin.org)

Nature. 2020 (August 19), "Progress report on the coronavirus pandemic". Volume 584 Issue 78821. Accessed July 15, 2022, https://www.nature.com/articles/d41586-020-02414-1

—. 2021. (May 4), "China's COVID vaccines are going global – but questions remain". Accessed Jun 15, 2022, https://www.nature.com/articles/d41586-021-01146-0

—. 2022 (December 9), "China is relaxing its zero-COVID policy: here's what scientists think". Accessed April 29, 2023, https://www.nature.com/articles/d41586-022-04382-0

Nature Briefing. 2023 (May 4), "Wuhan market samples fail to shed further light on COVID origins". Accessed May 6, 2023, https://www.nature.com/ articles/d41586-023-01483-2

NIH: National Institute of Allergy and Infectious Diseases. (Reviewed on March 21, 2022), COVID-19 Research at the Integrated Research Facility at Fort Detrick. Accessed April 10, 2023, https://www.niaid.nih.gov/research/covid-19-research-integrated-research-facility

Needham, Joseph (with the research assistance of Wang Ling), 1956, *History of Scientific Thought*. Vol. 2 in the *Science and Civilisation in China* series. Cambridge: Cambridge University Press

—. 2000, *Medicine, Science and Civilisation in China series*, Vol. 6, Part 6. Editor: Nathan Sivin, Cambridge: Cambridge University Press

Newsweek. 2020 (24 August), "JOE BIDEN WANTS A MASK MANDATE". Accessed August 12, 2021, https://www.newsweek.com/fact-check-mask-mandate-unconstitutional-1542465

Nice/National Institute for Health and Clinical Excellence. Accessed September 15, 2022, http://www.nice.org.uk/

Noble, Denis. 2006. *The Music of Life: Biology Beyond Dreams*, Oxford: Oxford University Press

Normile, Dennis. 2022 (1 March), "China quietly plans a pivot from 'zero COVID': Scientists are studying how to live with the virus while avoiding a crisis like in Hong Kong", *Science*, Vol 375, Issue 6584, 949. Accessed April 4, 2022, https://www. science.org/content/article/china-quietly-plans-pivot-zero-covid

Nozick, Robert. 1974, *Anarchy, State and Utopia*, New York: Basic Books.

O'Connor, J., and McDermott, I. 1997, *The Arts of Systems Thinking*. London: Thorsons

O'Connor, Timothy 2021 (Winter). "Emergent Properties", *The Stanford Encyclopedia of Philosophy* (Winter 2021 Edition), Edward N. Zalta (ed.). Accessed April 22, 2022, https://plato.stanford.edu/cgi-bin/encyclopedia/archinfo.cgi?entry=properties-emergent.

Oran, Daniel P., and Topal, Eric J. 2021 (May), "The Proportion of SARS-CoV-2 Infections That Are Asymptomatic: A Systematic Review". *Annals of Internal Medicine*: Vol 174, No 5. Accessed July 6, 2022, https://www.acpjournals.org/doi/full/10.7326/M20-6976?rfr_dat=cr_pub++0pubmed&url_ver=Z39.88-2003&rfr_id=ori%3Arid%3Acrossref.org

Our World In Data. 2023 (28 February), "China: Coronavirus Pandemic". Accessed February 28, 2023, https://ourworldindata. Org / coronavirus /country/china?country=~CHN

—. 2023. (April 26), "What is the cumulative number of confirmed cases? Accessed April 26, 2023, https://ourworldindata.org/covid-cases#what-is-the-cumulative-number-of-confirmed-cases; "What is the cumulative number of confirmed deaths?" Accessed April 26, 2023, https://ourworldindata.org/covid-deaths?country=IND~USA~GBR~CAN~DEU~FRA~CHN#what-is-the-cumulative-num

O'Rourke, Ciara. 2020 (18 September). "CDC Director Robert Redfield says healthy people should NOT wear masks". *PolitiFact*. Accessed August 8, 2021, https://www.politifact.com/factchecks/2020/sep/18/instagram-posts/cdc-director-says-healthy-people-should-wear-masks/ .

"Progress report on the coronavirus pandemic", *Nature* 2020 (19 August). Volume 584, Issue 7821, 325. Accessed January 24, 2022, https://www.nature.com /articles/ d41586-020-02414-1

Reuters. 2020 (4 September), "Fact check: Face masks being worn in China before COVID-19 doesn't prove they are ineffective". Accessed August 8, 2021, https://www.reuters.com/article/uk-factcheck-china-mask-covid-idUSKBN 25V1UR

"Role of Environmental Factors in Gene Expression", 2012, *Biotechnology Forums, COM*. Accessed May 28, 2022, https://www. biotechnology forums.com/thread-1798.html

Sachs, Jeffrey, Horton, Richard, Bagenal, Jessamy, Amor, Yanis Ben, Caman, Ozge Karadag, and Lafortune, Guillaume. 2020 (9 July), *The Lancet Commission on lessons for the future from the COVID-19 pandemic*. Accessed October 20, 2022, https://doi.org/10.1016/S0140-6736(20)3149-x ; https://www.thelancet.com/pdfs/journals/lancet/ PII S0 40-6736(22)01585-9.pdf

SAGE Report. 2022 (26 May), "Consensus statement on the association between the discharge of patients from hospitals and COVID in care homes". Accessed July 7, 2022, https://www.gov.uk/government/publications/the-association-between-the-discharge-of-patients-from-hospitals-and-covid-in-care-homes/consensus-statement-on-the-association-between-the-discharge-of-patients-from-hospitals-and-covid-in-care-homes

Schama, Simon. 2023 (May 25), *Foreign Bodies: Pandemics, Vaccines and the Health of Nations*, Simon & Schuster

Schulz, Bailey. 2021 (23 August), "CDC warns older adults, travelers in COVID high-risk groups not to take cruises, even if they're vaccinated", *USA Today*. Accessed September 21, 2022, https://eu.usatoday.com/story/travel/ cruises/2021/08/20/cruises-and-covid-19-cdc-updates-guidance-high-risk-travelers/8218346002/

Silverman, W. A. 1985, *Human Experimentation: a Guided Step into the Unknown,* Oxford: Oxford University Press

Sivin, Nathan. 1990, Science and Medicine in Chinese History. *Heritage of China: Contemporary Perspectives on Chinese Civilization*, ed, Paul Ropp. Berkeley: University of California Press

Sky News UK. 2020 (20 July), "Coronavirus: Anti-mask activists protest against order to wear face coverings". Accessed August 11, 2021, https://news.sky.com/story/coronavirus-anti-mask-activists-protest-against-order-to-wear-face-coverings-12032097

Sridhar, Devi. 2022, (14 July, 15 July and 22 July), "How Covid Changed Science. Three Episodes", Radio 4, BBC. Accessed August 19, 2022. https://BBC Radio 4 - How Covid Changed Science.

Stewart, G. T. 1968, "Limitations of the Germ Theory", *The Lancet*, Vol. 291 (7551), p. 1077-1081,

Stoneman, Justin. 2021 (17 July), "Cloth face masks are 'comfort blankets' that do little to curb Covid spread, Scientist warns", *The Telegraph*. Accessed August 12, 2021, https://www.telegraph.co.uk/news/ 2021/07/17/cloth-face-masks-comfort-blankets-do-little-curb-covid -spread/?WT.mc_id=tmgliveapp_iosshare_AxdbmR7tGYPz

Taylor, F. Kraűpl. 1979, *The Concept of Illness, Disease and Morbus*, Cambridge University Press,

Teller Report. 2020 (31 March), "Are all viruses "pathogenic"? Wrong!" Accessed March 11, 2022, https://Are all viruses "pathogenic"? wrong! - Teller Report

The British Medical Journal. 2021 (11 February), Editor's Choice. "Covid 19: Two million deaths, so what went wrong?" *British Medical Journal* 2021;372n393. Accessed October 16, 2022, http://doi.org/10.1136/bmj.n393; https:// www.bmj. com/ content/ 372/bmj.n393

The Guardian. 2022(29 December), "Why did China relax its Covid policy – and should we be worried". Accessed: April 30, 2023), https://www.theguardian.com/world/2022/dec/29/why-did-china-relax-its-covid-policy-and-should-we-be-worried#:~:text=After%20long%20 pursing%20a%20zero,including%20quarantine%20rules%20for%20travellers

The Harvard Crimson. 1952 (June17), "Class of 1927 Fails to Reproduce Itself, National Statisticians Claim". Accessed August 13, 2021, https://www.thecrimson.com/article/1952/6/17/class-of-1927-fails-to-reproduce/

The Intercept. 2023 (10 May), "THE RISE AND FALL OF THE RACCOON DOG THEORY OF COVID-19: Media reports created a false impression of a major breakthrough linking animals to Covid's origins". Accessed May 11, 2023, https://theintercept.com/ 2023/ 05/ 10/covid-pandemic-origin-raccoon-dog/

The Lancet. 2005 (October 22), "Nobel Prize winners Robin Warren and Barry Marshall". Accessed May 8, 2023, https://www.thelancet.com/ journals/lancet/article/PIIS0140-6736(05)67587-3/fulltext

The New York Times. 2023 (May 1), "In China, It's time to Splurge Again, and the Luxury Industry is Relieved". Accessed: May 3, 2023, https:/ /www.nytimes.com/2023/05/02/business/china-luxury-spending.html? campaign_id=51&emc=edit_mbe_20230503&instance_id=91636&nl= morning-briefing%3A-europe-edition&regi_id=161238284&segment _id=131964&te=1&user_id=373a935f3ce4812abad6007c0111ff79

—. 2023 (May 5), "W.H.O. ends Global Health Emergency Designation for Covid", Accessed: May 9, 2023, https://www.nytimes.com/2023/05/05/ health/covid-who-emergency-end.html?campaign_id=34&emc= edit_sc_20230509&instance_id=92112&nl=science-times&regi_id= 161238284&segment_id=132469&te=1&user_id=373a935f3ce4812 abad 6007c0111ff79

"To Mask or Not to Mask? CDC's Mixed Messages During the Pandemic" (GovExec Daily staff examines the pandemic response from the most-visible federal health agency) 2023 (25 January). Government Executive, Accessed: January 25, 2023, https://www.govexec.com/workforce/ 2023/01/mask-or-not-mask-cdcs-mixed-messages-during-pandemic/ 382161/

"The Sinovac-CoronaVac COVID-19 vaccine: What you need to know". 2022 (10 June), WHO. Accessed August 29, 2022, https://www.The Sinovac-CoronaVac COVID-19 vaccine: What you need to know (who.int)

"Timeline of Trump's Coronavirus Responses. 2022 (2 March)" Lloyd Doggett, US Representative, Blog Post. Accessed June 16, 2022, https:// doggett.house.gov/media/blog-post/timeline-trumps-coronavirus-responses

Van-Tam, Jonathan. 2021, (Three Lectures – RI 2021 Christmas Lectures) "Going viral: How Covid changed science forever – The Invisible enemy", The Royal Institute. Accessed February 11, 2022, https://www.rigb.org/explore-science/explore/video/going-viral-how-covid-changed-science-forever-invisible-enemy-2021

Victor, Daniel, Serviss, Lew, and Paybarah, Azi. 2020 (2 October), "In His Own Words, Trump on the Coronavirus and Masks", *The New York Times*. Accessed August 11, 2021, https://www.nytimes.com/ 2020/ 10/ 02/us/politics/donald-trump-masks.html

Wagner, Andreas. 2023 (6 April), *Sleeping Beauties: The Mystery of Dormant Innovations in Nature and Culture*, OneWorld Publications

Wang, Yuxin, Deng, Zicheng, and Shi, Donglu. 2021 (5 January), "How effective is a mask in preventing COVID-19 infection?" *Med. Devices Sens*. Accessed September 2, 2021, https://www.ncbi.nlm.nih.gov/pmc/articles/ PMC 78 83189/

Webb, Elizabeth. 2021 (9 June), "Coronavirus risk for older people", Age UK. Accessed July 10, 2022, https://www.ageuk.org.uk/discover/2020/06/coronavirus-risk-for-older-people-updated/

Wedgewood, Ralph. 2011, "Instrumental Rationality", *Oxford Studies in Metaethics,* R. Shafer-Landau (Ed.), Oxford: Oxford University Press, 280-309

WHO/World Health Organisation. 2020 (28 February), "Report of the WHO-China Joint Mission on Coronavirus Disease 2019 (COVID – 19)". Accessed January 31, 2022, https://www.who.int/ publications/ i/ item/report-of-the-who-china-joint-mission-on-coronavirus-disease-2019-(covid-19)

—. 2020 (4 April), Archived: "WHO Timeline – COVID-19". Accessed June 4, 2022, https://www.who.int/news-room/ detail/27-04-2020-who-timeline---covid-19

—. 2022 (5 May), "14.9 million excess deaths associated with the COVID-19 pandemic in 2020 and 2021". Accessed June 26, 2022, https: //www.who.int/news/item/05-05-2022-14.9-million-excess-deaths-were-associated-with-the-covid-19-pandemic-in-2020-and-2021

—. 2022 (11 August), "Tracking SARS-CoV-2 variants". Accessed September 12, 2022, https://www.who.int/activities/tracking-SARS-CoV-2-variants

Williams, Rose. 2021 (17 August), "36 parent advocacy groups reject forced masking in letter to Walz", *Alpha News*. Accessed August 17, 2021, http://36 parent advocacy groups reject forced masking in letter to Walz - Alpha News (alphanewsmn.com)

Wong, Chit Ming, Tsang, Hilda, Lai, Hak Kan, Thomas, G. Neil, Lam, Kin Bong, Chan, King Pan, Zheng, Qishi, Ayres, Jon G., Lee Siu Yin, Lam, Tai Hing, and Thach, Thuan Quoc. 2016. "Cancer Mortality Risks from Long-term Exposure to Ambient Fine Particles", *Cancer Epidemiology, Biomarkers & Prevention*, Volume 25, Issue 5, 1 May 2016. Accessed March 12, 2022, https://aacrjournals.org/cebp/article/25/5/839/71066/Cancer-Mortality-Risks-from-Long-term-Exposure-to

Woolf, Louis I and Adams, John. 2020, "The Early History of PKU" *International Journal of Neonatal Screen*, 2020 Sep; 6(3): 59. Accessed April 6, 2023, https://www.ncbi.nlm.nih.gov/pmc/articles/ PMC 7570 0 64/ ,

Worldometer. 2023 (29 January), "Reported Cases and Deaths by Country or Territory". Accessed January 31, 2023, https://www.worldometers.info/coronavirus/

Wulff, Henrik R. 1984, "The Causal Basis of the Current Disease Classification" *Health, Disease, and Causal Explanations in Medicine*, Eds. Lennart Nordenfelt. Dordrecht: D. Reidel Publishing Company, 169-177. Accessed 19/10/2022, https://link.springer.com/chapter/10.1007/978-94-009-6283-5_19

INDEX

H

I

J

L

M

R

S

T

U

V

W